This is a follow-up publication of the same text of
the book **Re-Member Africa**

www.re-memberafrica.org

The book cover: The painting is a very valuable
artwork from an anonymous African painter telling
the story of Africa in the last half millennium. The
right half has less mystery than the left.

Africa's Message to Obama

On why America's foreign policy on Africa should be centred on the accelerated political unification of the continent

Temi Metseagharun

iv

To you, SAK

CONTENTS

Introduction: The message

"Remember me . . . Save my soul," says Africa.
. . . and who knoweth whether thou art come to the kingdom for such a time as this? (Esther Chapter 4: 14).
O Barack, It is no coincidence that thou son of a full-blooded African is the current president of the United States of America.
Nobody said it will be easy to remember me . . . but at least we must start . . . you, given all your unique circumstances, must do this and give me my push and momentum . . .
"I was dismembered . . . and I am still bleeding," says Africa.
To re-member me is not to have me in your mind or memory, but to put my dismembered parts back together, O Barack.
To "Re-Member" Africa is to put her dismembered parts together genuinely in a political entity with strength and unity. United we stand, divided we fall. That political entity has already been born. Yes, it is the infantile and therefore weak African Union (AU) which now needs to be transformed into a truly democratic pan-African federal superstate, with an original and genuinely representative tribal congress and modern parliaments elected by the citizens of Africa – home and abroad – and a binding constitution for all states.
O Barack, no one is asking you or any other individual to solve the problems of a billion people in the whole continent of Africa. Indeed, you must be familiar with the following statements as premises:
"Africa's future is up to Africans . . . Africans must learn to solve their own problems by themselves . . . We cannot continue to infringe on the sovereignty of other countries . . . Africans must stop blaming colonialism of the past for the problems of the present"
Fine, but to forget the left hand of the past and then assume that decisions made within individual "states" in the continent will fix the problems is to naively work with the right hand alone . . . the human right hand of futuristic hopes and dreams. Here is the all-important question regarding the sovereign

1

countries of Africa: Infringement on the sovereignty of which countries? The countries or nations of the authentic tribes of the continent formed by their consent and voluntarily coming together? Or the "countries" imposed on the authentic nations by the Berlin Conference of 1884-1885? O Barack, it is a mistake to ask Africans to simply get on with the boundaries imposed on them, just as it is a mistake to assume that the effect of slavery is past, and that the past is always past, dead and buried. No. Not in the mind. Something else big, strong and good enough must emerge to lessen the negative effects of the past. Africa's future is up to which Africans? Which Africans must learn to solve their own problems by themselves? The extremely incompetent, psychopathically corrupt and self-serving Mugabes, Abachas, Gaddafis, Gbagbos, Mobutus, and other indigenous neo-colonialists of Africa who will never leave the political scene peacefully? Or the genuine and meek Africans including those in Diaspora with no voice such as the 5000 Nigerian doctors in the UK alone? With the power of incumbency and psychopathic corruption, the future of Africa is not up to the common people, but to indigenous neo-colonialist who were fortunate enough to be handed the geographical real estates of their erstwhile colonial masters. Oh no Barack, colonialism is not past, but was transformed in Africa and may remain so with new exploiters coming in to take advantage of the people, if the continent is not re-membered. Remembering Africa is the pan-Africanist position of greater unity amongst Africans with a union government, but one that grants greater autonomy to the numerous ethnic nations within their colonial boundaries. It is very much against any form of secession and the production of any more "countries" such as Eritrea and South Sudan, out of Africa.

What about people of African descent who have powerful voices? Will they simply claim to have African blood and not help the voiceless in their ancestral continent? As the European Diaspora helped Europe less than 100 years ago, so also, Africans in Diaspora should today, come to the aid of

Africa irrespective of their current citizenship. The core message is that for well over a century, the authentic peoples and voices of Africa have been ignored by fake nationalists (tribalists and indigenous neo-colonialists underneath) and the international community for the sake of convenience. The kind of convenience here is very much like calling people and places in Africa, new names that suit others such as foreign administrators or authors. 100 years ago Europe would rather deal with just one protectorate or "country" called Nigeria instead of 250 small ethic nations in the same geographical area. Indeed, most people outside Africa lump all the 54 countries in the continent and just talk about "Africa," so why not allow Africa to be one state? Nonetheless, we must not sacrifice authenticity for convenience. This is why within the proposed truly united continent, the authentic tribal or ethnic nations will be the federating units. This will allow the voices of the Ogonis, the Cabinda people, the Luos, the Hutus, the Thembu nation, the Itsekiris, the Igbos, and the other seemingly innumerable but authentic African nations to be heard, whilst retaining the colonial boundaries. There can be no true federalism within the boundaries of most of the current Europe-created colonial states, and with the way the politics of Africa is at the moment, true federalism can only be realised in a pan-African superstate. It is a mistake to force nations into any supposedly united political entity simply by human fiat, no matter how good the intention is. Yet, it is a strong pan-African superstate with one army that will obviate the need for foreign military intervention in African affairs. Yes, one professional 21st century army and not the useless or contemptible armies across Africa that recurrently seize the (colonial-boundary) state in unnecessary coups, make themselves instruments of despots, kill their own people and rape their own women!

If Nigerians are already calling on the African Court on Human and Peoples' Rights to address the failure of the state to provide primary education for citizens, then we can see how

3

a well-built pan-African superstate will guarantee rights and compel public office-holders and states to focus on their proper duties – instead of using the office for mainly personal ends as it is at the moment. We cannot turn back the hands of time, but those Africans, especially technocrats, who now claim to be educated and enlightened enough to see the bigger picture and the strength in diversity, must now use their intellectual prowess and creativity to create a new future for Africa that specifically excludes our current psychopathically corrupt and usually incompetent "leaders" by building a pan-African superstate big and diverse enough to be above racism, tribalism, and nepotism. A Pan-African superstate that is strong enough to eliminate the demon of psychopathic corruption and self-serving rulers; sophisticated and intellectually challenging enough to exclude half-educated politicians from government and to be united in spirit, truth and purpose enough to actually work in practice to ensure economic growth for the people. Yes, it is a challenge, but not for all Africans; just those who claim to understand the affairs of Africa.

Desperately needed foreign direct investments into Africa free of reciprocal corruption will be appropriately assured in Special Administrative Areas or regions of Africa under the superstate structure, built with long-term vision, competence and the benefit of the people at heart. Ultimately, the long hoped-for genuine economic growth in Africa without false starts and an end to the extreme poverty and widespread corruption in Africa will be achieved with the union government and the flourishing of the continent's authentic nations.

The African Diaspora, which includes you by the way, must rise up with one voice to unite the continent. You should be under understandable pressure to act, lest history be written that you were told, and you could have at least helped in starting the pan-African superstate and build U.S foreign policy for Africa on it, but you failed to, and then . . . your successor picked the idea up, and implemented it.

4

For if thou altogether holdest thy peace at this time, then shall
there enlargement and deliverance arise to the Jews (Africans)
from another place (China perhaps) . . . (Esther Chapter 4:
14).
America's foreign policy for Africa should now be centred on
the accelerated political unification of Africa, with the full
democratization and establishment of a pan-African superstate
out of the current infantile (weak) AU.

This is the message *from your forefathers on this side of the*
world. It is not an academic thesis rich in facts, figures, and
empirical data but it carries the weight of history, the blood of
Patrice Lumumba and the truth and spirit in the Bible. The
vessel: Dr Temi Metseagharun

Chapter 1

Who is the messenger?

As a junior doctor early in the year 2000, I remember walking into the office of Prof F. W Hickling, my supervising consultant and an Afro-Caribbean psychiatrist in the UK on a Wednesday morning. We were supposed to have a one hour session of clinical supervision.

"Last night, I don't know why, but I spent a lot of time thinking about you," he said.

Now, considering the length of time since this event I cannot remember every detail of our subsequent conversation, but he seemed to give me the impression that his spirit was disturbed to a point where he could not sleep initially. I was immediately concerned; fearing for my clinical work as a first year trainee psychiatrist. Fear turned to feeling flattered, when the subsequent conversation changed to the subject of Africa and how educated Nigerians hold so much hope for black Africans and the black race. I did not initially share his views on black and African affairs, but the first message from Africa *("Remember me . . . save my soul")* came from him to me and has never left my soul. In subsequent meetings, he told me of the "dismembering of Africa" and how the solution to the problems of Africa must be about "re-membering" a dismembered body.

"Interesting," I said to myself at the time without paying much attention. Besides, he said he was going to write a book with the title *Remembering Africa* and so, I felt I should wait for the publication of the book. It seems that was not to be, as instead 11 years on, here I am as his former pupil writing you this letter in the form of a book.

My name is Dr Temi Metseagharun and I believe I could be accurately portrayed as *"an average African living in the UK."* I was born and raised in Nigeria until age 25 when I left for the UK with one eye on furthering my postgraduate studies and another eye, like most African migrants, on the supposedly greener pastures outside of Africa. The question however is why should you or any other political decision maker listen to me – an ordinary or average African - as a credible messenger? Calling myself "average" is not an attempt to come across as modest, but a reflection of the reality of the problems of Africa including "brain drain" where the average African living abroad is generally literate and more educated than her average counterpart back home - having voted with her feet. This is simply a form of visa-related selection bias, which means that the average African in the UK or indeed the USA is likely to be a medical doctor or another professional whose professional skill was not planned for or valued enough by the self-serving autocrats who couldn't care less if they left the country for greener pastures or not. But what has an average African living in the UK or the USA got to say about Africa? Should we not be consulting African leaders and recognised intellectuals on the subject of Africa's development? My answer is NO! If they had the answers, competence, honesty or political will, then Africa will not be where she is today. As a matter of fact you and the United States Government have an army of sincere messengers as revealed by wikileaks. I speak largely with my experience of Nigeria, but Ambassadors John Campbell and Robin Sanders know more than I or the average Nigerian about the incompetence and corruption of the "leaders" of our "country" Nigeria. With those leaked diplomatic cables, it is clear that you already know of the extent of the problem and I really do not need to tell you much. As an authentic messenger of Africa however, I offer you a spiritual cable for the solution. For the solution is not necessarily known by those who know the extent of the problem. As a doctor, this is a familiar scenario to me. The pathologist has no cure for the physician's challenges. My focus on Nigeria is not parochial, but reflects the importance of the geographical area called Nigeria and the great hope for black Africa that the people -

8

the salt - in the area carry. *But if the salt have lost his savour, wherewith shall it be salted?* - Matthew 5:13. In the following paragraphs, I will digress a bit, but it is about putting the messenger into context.

Many writings such as those of the likes of Martin Meredith (the author of *The State of Africa,* 2005), Paul Collier (author of *The Bottom Billion,* 2008), Vijay Mahajan (author of *Africa Rising,* 2009), Dambisa Moyo (author of Dead Aid, 2009), William Easterly (author of The *White Man's Burden,* 2006) and even Chinua Achebe (the author whose book, *Things Fall Apart,* Nelson Mandela read in prison and found as medicine for his soul; Nelson Mandela said Achebe had "brought Africa to the rest of the world" and described him as "the writer in whose company the prison walls came down") all give good insight and probable solutions to the problems of Africa. However, with the internet and the evolution of blogs, the uncensored opinions of the average African can be explored and found to be more insightful than any book. Sadly, no powerful political decision maker has time to read millions of comments on the problems of Africa. You should listen to the average African, and why he is abroad - Europe and the USA most especially - and not in his native land today. One most insightful review on Amazon.com by A. O Akemu on Paul Collier's book is as follows (excerpts):

He (Professor Collier) *also rightly points out that in a number of bottom-billion countries, there are courageous men and women, who are working hard at reforming their economies. He names a few of them like Nigeria's Ngozi Okonjo-Iweala and Charles Soludo. Professor Collier notes that these brave people deserve support. So true!*

Furthermore, he criticizes aid policy as had been administered to date. Aid has not worked and for good reason: it has been badly administered and done with the heart and not the head. As one who is sceptical of the arguments of both the aid-loving left and the aid-bashing right, I was pleased to read how Collier strikes a balance between both camps. His point: aid

9

does not have to be given to poor countries as a sop for colonialism. It must be committed, targeted and given for over a decade to post-conflict societies.

Professor Collier observes that Africa has the largest number of landlocked countries in the world. According to him, "...The international system should not have let them become economic entities in the first place..." Well, that's putting a gloss on the issue here. Why not call a spade a spade? The reason why there are so many landlocked countries in Africa is colonialism. Countries like Chad and Burkina Faso were carved up as French zones of influence in 1888 and remain so till this day. The Professor does not even mention the "C" word. In his book, he asks us to get over it and move on as these countries are here to stay. True, but this is an injustice to the readers, who may not understand that most African countries are not really "nations".

Reading the book, you'll get the impression that Africans just squandered the heaven-sent aid from the West in the last 50 years. The truth is slightly more complex: there was the added complication of the Cold War, which was anything but cold in the Third World. Indeed, Africa and Latin America were key frontlines in the Cold War. It is in Africa, for example, that the US supported unsavoury dictators like Mobutu Sese-Seko and Jonas Savimbi's UNITA, leading them to commit the most egregious crimes against their own people. Professor Collier does not tell this side of the story well.

In response to, and agreeing almost entirely with A. O Akemu, Dreamer, a very insightful commentator who interestingly, but not helpfully chose to make his very intelligent views with a bit of sarcasm known under a pseudonym, had the following to say (excerpts):

The Niger Delta constitutes one of the biggest contributors to global warming on planet earth because we have no idea of what to do with the Natural Gas that is a by-product of oil exploration and recovery. We flare it (flare means "to set fire to, in order to burn" i.e. it's burning as I speak). The carbon dioxide thus generated is a greenhouse gas.

I do not presuppose the heat generated from such senseless activities on a truly hellish scale will help in cooling down the planet. The devil must have a most comfortable living environment in that Niger Delta, because hell is very hot according to the Bible. Maybe that's why Nigeria is so upside down, his activities are becoming too wide ranging over there. The price of this gas is for evermore galloping upwards and onwards and never comes down. Have you ever witnessed your British Gas bill falling? No! It's always progressing in leaps and bounds. Why don't we just say, "Let us be slaves, Amen."

Remember that Nigeria is not at all land locked. We have a very long coast line formerly known as the "Slave Coast" (the Slave Coast starts somewhere around Ghana and ends somewhere after the Bight of Bonny), where we used to export slaves from en masse, with the help of the Portuguese and the British.

There was the Ivory Coast, the Gold and the "Slave Coast". I wish I was from Botswana. They have no coast. They are landlocked.

I recently found out that "Escravos" is a Portuguese word for slave. I never knew. I thought Escravos was a Mid-Western Nigerian word. Now, there is a tributary of the River Niger in the Niger Delta, a river known as Escravos. Many people will have heard of Oil and Gas projects around Escravos in Nigeria.

It all came home to me. I mean the meaning of the phrase "he's been sold down the river". It's a Nigerian phrase. It means "to be cheated out of something" nowadays.
  - Dreamer (Pseudonym of an Amazon blogger)

Most views or statement expressed in blogs and public commentary -including the ones above -may not be entirely correct and can be faulted, but this is not a significant issue considering the need for the commoner to express his democratic rights and say. Neither I nor the average blogger is ashamed of expressing a view that may turn out to be erroneous. We are after the truth, not bits of facts. This position is safer than entrusting our salvation to the single mind of an aristocrat (you know what I mean; that some expert – or financial adviser - may simply be highly knowledgeable for a world that is no more and cannot recognise innovation). I, as a messenger of Africa, have certainly not read enough reviews and blogs, but would still like to attempt to embody and personify the blogosphere of the average African living abroad. By coincidence or spiritual design, my ancestral homeland happens to be the very "Escravos" with Oil and gas projects that Dreamer wrote about and unknown to the world, a land of so much tears and blood including that of my gentle father (may his soul rest in peace). For me, a part of the statement of A.O Akemu ["*In his book, he asks us to get over it* (colonialism and by default slavery) *and move on as these countries are here to stay. True, but this is an injustice to the readers, who may not understand that most African countries are not really "nations".*] on the opinion of Professor Collier, hit the nail on the head with regard to this letter to you O Barak Obama. There is a real continent –Africa – and the "states" that make up Africa are artificial and basically an accident of European history, and therefore made of rotten foundation (the Berlin conference) that can hardly and should not be built on. Nonetheless, all accidental histories including the natural history of biological evolution, are here to stay as are the problems due to biological history; genetic disorders and inflammation of a useless organ such as the appendix resulting in potentially fatal appendicitis.

In 1979 as a 7 year-old Nigerian primary school pupil, I was told (and genuinely believed as most children would) that I was amongst the leaders of tomorrow. In 1999 (20 years later),

Nigeria took a metaphorical 20 years backward step by selecting and imposing the same Head of State of 20 years earlier in a sham election – the cornerstone of sham democracy in Africa. With the imagination of a child, I never stopped dreaming of a greater Africa, and as an 11 year old in 1983, I stayed all night listening to election results that even as a child I knew were doctored. That was when I first shed tears for Africa. I look back now and wonder why I was so keen on politics at that age.

As a 14 year old high school student, 3 of my classmates and I went for a "National Young Scientist Competition" and were sensitized to what I thought was our great potential to be really helpful to our world through academic abilities with more "leaders of tomorrow" talk by enthusiastic teachers and even the television workers we met.

Next came the university environment from age 15 in 1987 to age 21 where I faced my own identity crisis – as some, if not most teenagers do – in medical school. I have to admit that there was little modelling from national political figures as late 1983 until 1999 saw Nigeria being ruled by self-serving military dictators deceiving themselves and the public about governance. The truth of course is that everywhere in the world, anything but the briefest of military governments can be nothing but the preservation of the interests of a few elite disguising as government. This military period saw the government closing down universities for long periods because of absolutely justified students' unrest. This was the period that a brigadier ridiculously became the "sole administrator" or de-facto vice chancellor of a Nigerian University. For my political interests, I got to the position of secretary general of the college of medicine student's association, and no further. However, my short student political career opened my eyes to the power of modelling. Even in the student union, students had learnt from the rulers of the state and began to embezzle student union funds. To the credit of the student union government administration that I was a part of, and to the young medical students in politics at

13

the time, we succeeded in prosecuting our former student leaders and got them to return stolen funds. I go into my background because I have become aware that this negative modelling has sunk so deep that it has become the norm even amongst lecturers and so-called intellectuals. Everyone, but very few committed individuals have joined the corruption bandwagon for the sake of "survival." This, although quite sad, was explained as a "necessity" where people must live first and then combat corruption later and that had I not left the country 13 years earlier, I certainly will not be writing this "righteous letter." I have to say at this point that I am not simply one of those "Nigerians in Diaspora" who sit in the comfort of their homes abroad and criticise the effort that those who remained behind are making to lift the country out of poverty and bad governance.

I have acted on the urgings of the late Gani Fawehinmi of Nigeria to *"stand for what is right, even if you are standing alone."* I organised and paid for a supposedly annual "National Anti-corruption Essay competition" in 2003 and 2004 in Nigeria. I look back and wonder why I had done it, as even my close associates were not particularly supportive and the minister of Education at the time did not respond to a letter I had written to him. I suppose living in the U.K and seeing my patients consistently having responses to their letters driven by illness, made me to imagine that a "government" in Africa will bother to respond to a letter from an ordinary person. I also forgot that the "government" of Nigeria at the time, and as the product of sham democracy, was unlikely to respond to constructive suggestions from ordinary people, but I certainly got an enthusiastic response from the public including one newspaper editor. This has taught me that the people always respond to, and debate the burning issues of the day, but with sham governments and establishments, such debates are usually ignored. I now feel a strong need to communicate with you as the voice of the silent majority, and as one of the supposed political leaders of tomorrow now leading a struggle for hearts and minds on the true nature of

14

the problem of Africa. My hope (remember your campaign posters) therefore is that you Barack Obama and all your supporters will not ignore my letter.

It cannot be informative if we listen to those who had benefitted, and continue to benefit from the status quo; more like listening to Hosni Mubarak on 10th of February 2011. Therefore as a messenger I would say that we should listen to the honest opinions and statements of the refugees. I have been privileged and unfortunate at the same time to witness the political problems of my part of Africa from a relatively close range. I came over to the UK in early 1998 for postgraduate education, full of hope and promises as a 25 year-old doctor. My father S.A.K Metseagharun had made a similar journey 26 years earlier and indeed he was in the UK when I was born in Nigeria. He returned promptly to Nigeria after his diploma in overseas income taxes, and served the government and people of Delta state of Nigeria for 27 years in total before retiring as the Chairman/Sole Administrator of Delta State Board of Inland Revenue in 1997. He was among the few who sat on millions of dollars of government money and chose not to embezzle. I know this because I got real education and no inherited cash from him. It is worth stating that Delta State of Nigeria as an oil-producing state has a lot of money that was, and is still being embezzled. To give you an insight into the thieving and embezzlement going on in this Delta State of Nigeria (my supposed "state" within a supposed federation), it is interesting to note that a former governor in the same state that my father served for 27 years, is currently – as I write you this letter – on remand in a London prison and on trial on several counts related to alleged criminal activities. Back home in Nigeria, this ex-governor, James Ibori, was a king maker who contributed to "making" the late Umaru Yar'Adua president of Nigeria as evidenced by the appointment of Ibori's former commissioner for finance, David Edevbie, as Yar' Adua's Principal Private Secretary. Ibori had been charged to court in Nigeria's Kangaroo judicial system and acquitted of 70 counts related to theft. Prior to his

15

extradition to the UK from Dubai, his wife, concubine, sister and lawyer had all been found guilty of various charges related to theft. This is the on-going story of a state's "governor" . . . and with well-known criminals controlling the state. What can the people expect? We, the voiceless people have to rely on our ex-colonial master, Great Britain, to save us from thieves, just like France rescued Ivory Coast from Gbagbo and as the international community is doing for Libya as Gaddafi is bent on destroying all his people for his own ends, if that is what it takes to remain in office. There is no hope for the people of Africa when criminals have seized the state, and this is the context from which I am now writing and advocating a re-building of Africa with the exclusion of thieves and self-serving half-educated miscreants.

What happens to honest men and people of integrity in a criminals-controlled state? In my father's case, he was murdered – tortured to death – by his relations on 23rd September 1998, less than 2 years after retiring and barely 8 months into my stay in the UK. His killers, who are well known, since they are relations of his, are driving their flashy cars on the streets along which he was killed. Some of them are "advisers" to the state "governor" and not surprising, "friends" of the oil companies including the good U.S. company called Chevron. I will state at this point that I do not believe that Chevron in the U.S. is aware of some of the goings-on in Nigeria, and from my own family relationship with the company we have for long accepted Chevron as a benefactor. However, one of Chevron's supposedly innovative community development councils in the Niger Delta or "global MOU" was chaired by someone on trial for the murder and torture referred to above. Of course, I write as an insider and relative of both the deceased and the accused. It is not the investor's fault that the land they are investing in is controlled by criminals. I need not say much about Delta State as the leaked diplomatic cables contain enough about the state's previous governor and the Nigerian "judiciary."

The Nigerian judiciary that the messenger has witnessed is such that the guilty and the most dangerous to society are routinely granted bail for cash, innocent people are thrown in prison "awaiting trial" for several years (up to 15 years in one case), and the Supreme Court subverts justice at the request of a traditional ruler. It is amazing when Nigerian newspapers from time to time, report a supposedly caring judge releasing prisoners "awaiting trial." The news is not about the judge, but of a rotten and shambolic judiciary. I suppose this story is not a strange human story, but I have seen a system that is so rotten and I have smelt it from so close a range that it is understandable why I cannot have faith in these remnants of our colonial and slave trade-related contraption mistaken for a state. According to a Nigerian pundit what we are seeing in the system amounts to a *malodorous saga cum gargantuan gaga.* It is not an exaggeration to state that all arms of government in Nigeria are a complete sham; for the essence of a sham is in its looking like the real thing. The more it looks like the real thing, the more it is a sham; but in the end, a sham is a sham. It was in the process of setting up and running a non-governmental organisation or charitable foundation in my father's name, to address some of the relevant, but intractable issues that I improved my understanding of the international nature of Africa's problems. In my family's specific case, the presence of petroleum in our homeland of the Niger Delta – Escravos to be more specific – brought in foreign exploiters who in all honesty were exploiting oil, not the people initially. All that soon changed and the politics of oil began to take its toll and my father was killed over the crumbs of oil money falling on our oil-rich community land. The full story of oil, tears and blood in the Niger Delta as it affected the Metseagharuns will form a book, but it may be of interest to note that 12 years following my father's death, juju-worshipping individuals have taken over the administration of our local affairs. The metaphorical 20 years backward step for Nigeria in 1999 is not the only clear example. My ancestral homeland of Ugborodo (now called Escravos – the Portuguese

17

word for "the slaves") is where Chevron has its estimated $10 billon Escravos Gas To Liquid (EGTL) project. A few miles away from this project is a shrine for juju worship and occult practices that were the norm pre-colonisation. It is interesting to read Captain Alain Boisragon's description of my people's Juju worship over 110 years ago, indicative of our stagnation:

Although the languages are different, the manners and customs of the different tribes in the Protectorate are much the same. The great Mohammedan invasion, which came down from the north and founded the Hausa States, stopped short at the River Benué, the big confluent of the Niger, and never reached the country now under the Protectorate, so that it is still the land of Juju. Juju here is everything, religion, superstition, custom, anything.

Interestingly, despite the billions of dollars of investments in the Escravos area, not many people live there permanently. Is this evidence of state failure or a very bad case of corporate social irresponsibility? Who is to blame for the zero investments on true infrastructure which would have drawn the locals, tourists and other people to the beautiful mangrove swamp land, wild life and beaches that are the future economic potential for the people after the oil is exhausted, without irreversibly damaging the environment?

Bearing the issue of faulty (King Leopold II-related) foundations in the nationhood of several African "countries," and now, the power of incumbency in mind, how could we bring in progress, development and true freedom to Escravos? Should the United States government and the oil companies harden their consciences, by taking the oil from my land, colluding with the corrupt few in positions of authority and allowing some juju-worshiping people to impose their primitive ways on the rest of us? This question does not imply that our salvation is ultimately in the hands of foreign governments alone, but without France Gbagbo will still be one of two "presidents" of the Ivory Coast and without NATO Gaddafi would have murdered thousands of his people in order to remain in power. The point from this messenger is

that a stronger AU will remove the need for "foreign intervention" in African affairs in so many ways. There are some unique cultural problems that no intervention from outside can affect; and you probably don't want to hear of superstitious practises such as burning actual $1 million (UDS) cash with the faces of United States presidents to ashes in the Niger Delta and using the ashes dissolved in water to have a bath. Guess what this bath is supposed to achieve? Political power is the answer according to the reports.
Who can help individuals with such depth of superstition? Oh no, not even you Barack. As a people, we deserve to be supported to prevent such superstitious individuals from running our local and national affairs. The sad story is that they do in Nigeria and the ambitions of good people may be thwarted when they are required by those already in positions of authority to partake in occult practices before they will be enabled. You should listen to the voice of the authentic African in deciding U.S. foreign policy for Africa. I am the authentic voice of Africa. My background and current observations will naturally cause anyone in my position, and anyone who really cares to think quite deeply. Witnessing the political problems of my part of Africa from a very close range means that when I make certain statements, I make them from real life experience, and not just from what is written in a bestseller. Some of my fellow "Nigerians" have estimated that with "*the obstacle of incumbency*," where incompetent office holders tend not to leave office at any cost when due, it may take 5 generations (200 years) for Africa to be at par with the rest of the world. NO! I say, and this is why I have to convey this message to you.

Back to the person of Dr Temi Metseagharun, I will state early in this letter that my holding on to my tribal identity may be seized upon by "Nigerians" negatively as "tribalism" which is inimical to "nation building." Yes, I am an Itsekiri man, but like my grandfather, I was made a "Nigerian" as part of the collective delusion of a sham state. I identify with my father's

19

line, but being an Itsekiri could be through either parent. There is, as a matter of fact, no "pure Itsekiri." I do not believe in genetic or ethnic purity and to give a hint on my tribal/ethnic associations, I'll say that it is interesting to note that my children now have Itsekiri, Benin, Isoko, Scottish, Yemeni, Algerian and Moroccan bloods as far as we are aware . . .but are British by birth and current upbringing!

My being born and raised in Africa and my observation of events in Africa have turned me from a standard UK National Health Service psychiatrist to more of a philosopher-psychiatrist, writer and social entrepreneur. It seems like I am alone, but I'm not. Those who stand for what is right seemingly alone and in private, stand together in the sprit realm that knows no distance. It is this collective spirit that has made me a mouthpiece for the rest. If I don't do it, who will? I have asked myself. Professionally, I remain committed to mental health and my book *ABC of the Mind (Author House 2008)*, promises happiness and fulfilment to readers. I have a special interest in "The Spirituality of Psychiatry" and run a research project with the same theme. Most of my writings and meditation revolve around the "meaning of life," for what is mental illness if not the pain of living and the lack of meaning to a human life? But then, what gives meaning to human life if not self-determination and a sense of belonging? Mental health and politics go together.

I find myself explaining that my being a psychiatrist with personal experience of the problems of Africa puts me uniquely in a position to come up with the ideas for which I now have the commitment to turn into action. In terms of my credibility – and those of others like me – to handle this matter, it is relevant to note that I was one of the *"child leaders of tomorrow"* that bad governance, nepotism, wickedness, despotism and corruption in a sham state never allowed to appropriately serve his "country."

Furthermore, in terms of national service, it is worth noting that Nigeria has a National Youth Service Corps, under which I served between 1995 and 1996 as a medical officer. New graduates under this programme are required to serve outside their home states as a means of cementing the country's unity by exposing its leaders of tomorrow to other parts of the vast country. Sadly, at the point of the first draft of this letter, 10 corps members from southern Nigeria were reportedly killed in northern Nigeria in post-election violence. One can only imagine the grief and devastation of the families who have spent decades raising and educating their child to graduate level . . . only for their dreams to be shattered in an attempt to build a non-existent nation. What sort of country will brutally kill its youths whose services are specifically designed to unite the "nation"? Post-election violence and other ethnicity-driven carnage in Africa are the direct result of false nationhood. Economic development in such circumstances can only be by chance if the whole continent is not re-membered with the authentic nations as the units. This is the message and I am the messenger of Africa still in captivity and mental slavery . . . and by the rivers of Babylon there we sat down, and yea we wept when we remembered Zion (Africa). I am weeping, and I cannot sing in this letter, but songs of Africa have been in the air for centuries. The need for Africa to unite politically had been in the air even before "independence" was granted to previous colonies. Now is the time and I was raised with unique circumstances specifically to convey this message to you.

Chapter 2

The problems of Africa: Where can we start?

"In my mind, there are two parts to the story of the African peoples ... the rain beating us obviously goes back at least half a millennium. And what is happening in Africa today is a result of what has been going on for 400 or 500 years, from the "discovery" of Africa by Europe, through the period of darkness that engulfed the continent during the trans-Atlantic slave trade and through the Berlin Conference of 1885. That controversial gathering of the leading European powers, which precipitated the "scramble for Africa," we all know took place without African consultation or representation. It created new boundaries in ancient kingdoms, and nation-states resulting in disjointed, inexplicable, tension-prone countries today"

- Chinua Achebe (Author of Things fall apart)

In the preceding chapter I mentioned that there are several books on the problems of Africa and "the problem with Africa," all explaining why a continent of 1 billion human beings continue to suffer in the midst of plenty and in the most prosperous time of all human history. I cannot go into repeating what has been well described in several books, but it is relevant to ask exactly the same questions that Dambisa Moyo asked:
Why is it that Africa, alone among the continents of the world, seems to be locked into a cycle of dysfunction? Why is it that out of all the continents of the world Africa seems unable to convincingly get its foot on the economic ladder? Why in a recent survey did seven out of the top ten 'failed states' hail from the continent? Are Africa's people universally more

23

incapable? Are its leaders generally more venal, more ruthless, more corrupt? Its policy-makers more innately feckless? What is it that holds it back, that seems to render it incapable of joining the rest of the globe in the twenty-first century?

Moyo, a fellow African and a contrast in the non-African white male dominated public debate about Africa's economic problems, blames foreign aid; *"The answer has its roots in aid."* She says with good justification especially in terms of pointing out western aid involving *"I'll pay myself to help you"* type of help to a dying patient (my interpretation). In my medical world, she is saying that the disease is basically iatrogenic. . . . that is, this kind of headache is a side effect of paracetamol. No, it's not that simplistic, for there was a disease well before an unhelpful cure was experimented, but true that there is no point giving paracetamol for a brain tumour. I was immediately reminded of my psychologist colleague's story of how his Australian parents literally drank the fortunes – millions of dollars – of his Australian grandparents. Should we blame the availability of generally helpful medicines and psychoactive substances such as alcohol (foreign aid)? Or, should we blame the unavailability of an effective means of control (lack of protective international charters for preventing the exploitation of Africa and preventing corruption by African rulers) of such medicines? For those who seek a single answer to complex and multiple questions, the *answer has its roots in the history of the sham states of Africa.*

My mission in this letter remains the message for the solution and not a repetition of the descriptions of the problem. Some people frown at the bad image of Africa and a tendency for Africans and Western news media to feed this bad image. Well, Barack, I tell you compared to other parts of the world, Africa's current state is worse than the image. It is really bad. That is the simple truth. It is the complacency of the world and ignorance of how bad things really were that led to the 1994 genocide in Rwanda! As I write this letter to you O Barack,

24

Libya and Ivory Coast are desperately relying on foreign help to save them from their own "leaders," and both countries for decades were seemingly stable and prosperous. Others including the elephant – Nigeria – are bubbling underneath. Pockets of improvement and unsustainable growth should not distract anyone from the fact that overall, things are relatively worse than they were in Africa just prior to independence going by several measures of human progress. In all the accounts, opinions and arguments, the two hands of man and his 10 fingers – main villains – cannot escape blame for the mess. What we have witnessed in Africa over the last half millennium is an unnatural evolution that must be fixed by the same human hands. There is guidance on what is not cut out of human hands, but we'll have to wait until the next chapter.

The left human hand of the past
We can all research Africa's history and without too much revisionism the 5 fingers will be appreciated as follows:

1. **The slave trade and its demographic and socio-cultural catastrophe:** The slave trade may have done most of the damage to sub-Saharan Africa, not the more recent emigration of Africa's intelligentsia. The slave trade's impact on the continent is grossly underestimated! Just like no one really knows the losses recorded due to the destruction of the rain forests, so also, the losses of human traits and abilities during the slave trade are not really known. I honestly cannot tell whether or not this trade made the indigenous Africans extremely wicked and superstitious with their customs and traditions, or the customs facilitated the trade; but the history is undisputed that Africans sold their own people and "the other tribe" into slavery, killed people to bury their kings and killed twins. Now, their modern

25

incarnates stash away billions of dollars in foreign bank accounts whilst their fellow Africans die of starvation. Three hundred years of the trans-Atlantic slave trade altered the demographics and destroyed the natural path of native Africans' social evolution. More of this will be delved into later. We cannot imagine what 300 years of inter-tribal wars and kidnappings did to ancient African kingdoms. When the British entered the ancient Benin Kingdom in 1897, it was nothing compared to what the Portuguese and Dutch described 300 years earlier. The magnificent city with high earthen walls, broad roads and a king on horseback were nowhere to be found, but replaced by human sacrifices everywhere, according to the 1897 report by the British. Unless the tales and drawings of the Benin Kingdom of the 15th and 16th centuries were fabrications, then the slow but destructive effect of the slave trade must have been catastrophic. In terms of the magnificence of 300 years earlier, only the ancient art works, now scattered all over Europe , survived the period of slavery, it seems. This is really sad as it almost provides proof that Africa had been declining for 300 years before the Berlin Conference!

2. **Imperialism:** This refers to those who for whatever reason, choose to rule others. In this process began the phenomenon of *"taking from home and stashing away from home".* Considering this, the Belgian King Leopold II must be exhumed to pay reparations to the AU and not to "The Democratic republic of Congo", his private real estate colony that was never, and is still not a nation, like other "mere geographical

26

entities" masquerading as nations and having embassies all over the world and seats at the UN. There is no point repeating the story of the scramble for Africa, but one thing is clear from the history: most of the schizophrenic "countries" of Africa today are the children of Europe. I'm sorry mum, I am your child, and you raised me to become who I am today, despite the "independence" you gave to me at age 18. It is unfair to ask me to build a house that I know nothing about its planning (for whatever purpose) and architectural design. Worse still, is to ask a group of architects to continue from where another stopped with the later having a different vision from the former. Surely a re-start from scratch will be best!

3. **Human greed:** Refers to those who have modernised the very same *"taking from home and stashing away from home"* in the form of safe havens for stolen wealth and mineral exploitation with no genuine regard for the people of the land. Imperialism would not have been a bad thing had greed not been part of the equation. The greedy have been and still remain the partners of villain numbers 1 and 2. So, Switzerland, Shell and a few other mineral exploiting companies must attend a New Berlin Conference on how the EU, China and the USA must fund the AU's childhood and youth, and help solve some human population explosion and migration problems in the process.

4. **The cold war:** Those who fought their proxy wars in Africa. There is no need to explain further as the history is clear and those whose puppets killed and

maimed Africans must now own up to it. Now is the
time to fight a new proxy war of investments into
Africa through the AU; perhaps with new sides.
There are Special Administrative Regions and
continental roads such as the one from Cape Town to
Cairo to be built, African internal markets and trade
to be developed, hydroelectric power to be sourced
from the River Congo and several 21st century
continental cities to be built from scratch across the
continent – to help stem migration to Europe.

5. **Guilty, but pretentious bystanders:** Those who
   have sat, and continue to sit in the comfort of their
   homes, offices and cars not caring that their comfort
   may be partly bought with the tears and blood of
   people in a distant land. Voltaire's story of Candide
   pictures finger number 5 very clearly when Candide
   came across a Negro in a Dutch colony with one
   hand, one leg and a rag for clothing. The Negro's
   response: "When we work at the sugar canes," the
   slave explains, "and the mill snatches hold of a
   finger, they cut off a hand; and when we try to run
   away, they cut off a leg . . . . This is the price at
   which you eat sugar in Europe."

The Right Human Hand of the future

Africa's history is full of revisionism but there is no doubt that
that we are where we are primarily as the result of decisions
made outside the continent. To assume that decisions within
the continent will fix the present problems is to work naively
with the right hand alone . . . the human right hand of futuristic
hopes and dreams. The right hand is necessarily abstract and

therefore a thing of the mind . . . and perhaps where the opinions of Dr Temi may be seen to be more valid. This right hand has already been applied in Africa and indeed its failure so far had made it sometimes indistinguishable from the left hand, because the past is not really past. O Barack, what is the future if not history that is not yet written? O yes! Those that attempted to write the future history of Africa (see chapter 4) actually started in the mid-19th century and from there on we can see the 5 fingers of the right human hand as follows:

1. **Political philosophy:** Politics according to Will Durant is the study of ideal social organisation. It is not, as one might suppose, the art and science of capturing and keeping office. So, what kind of political philosophy applied during the Berlin Conference? I'll leave that for European historians to tell. Clearly, Africa's numerous pre-colonial monarchies were made irrelevant by imperialism, although a lot of the kings did not realise this. The original monarchies as exemplified by the Swazi king have little beyond relics of history and culture to demonstrate in the modern political arena, unless they are modernised. Collectively, we had no specific political philosophy, but the *Europeanisation of Africa* agenda seemed to offer an ideal social organisation to begin with, but with political changes elsewhere in the world, imperialism had to give way to independence and something else as the core political operating system. This was the beginning of the manifestation of Africa's political and economic schizophrenia! With the colonial "countries" lacking depth in terms of political and economic philosophy, democracy was the obvious choice as an operating system. In Nigeria democracy post-independence

immediately turned to "Demo-Crazy" or the demonstration of craze according to the African philosopher-musician Fela Anikulapo-Kuti. Nigeria's political schizophrenia soon led to the genocide of the Biafran war less than 7 years into "independence." Fela then asked, if it is not "craze", why is it in Africa? This is not to say that democracy is not suitable for Africa. For example some pundits talk about a "benevolent dictatorship," but how can you "democratise" or change a country without first changing the people's beliefs (right finger number 2)? The political philosophy (perhaps none, but human greed) that drove the Berlin Conference left a vacuum at independence which the right middle finger (number 3 – economic philosophy) took advantage of, leading at least in part to the very hot cold war – communism versus capitalism – of tears, blood and wickedness in Africa. Indeed the average human being uses the first 3 fingers to write, so how can we write a future with such faulty fingers? The truth of a "very hot cold war" in Africa is proof of political madness in Africa. There is no surprise here given the foundations of the "countries" whose political constitutional make up (not the biological constitutional make up or genes of the people) destined them for a developmental disorder, similar to the biological schizophrenia of human beings.

2. **The beliefs of the people:** The beliefs, attitude, culture, customs or traditions of people all over the world determine their political philosophy and ultimately who becomes their leader – unless they are conquered as it happened with colonialism. Sadly,

science has not given us a good understanding of how beliefs are formed in the brain and how deep down, delusions spring out of a seemingly normal brain. What we ordinary call "belief" is the subjective definition of reality and its spectrum spans the perception of other psychological entities such as emotions, urges, desire, attitude and even instincts – the software of the human brain. There is however no doubt that most people's beliefs are simply the reflection of their cultural environment and individual history. Bearing this in mind, it can be seen that only systematic and deliberate education and training can shift the individual from the vicarious learning that the environment offers. Sadly, the colonial masters did not stay long enough to educate the people and eliminate tragic customs such as juju worship and other occult rituals that have now morphed into the "psychopathic corruption" demonstrated by African political office holders of today who have perfected *the art and science of capturing and keeping office.* In rejecting an offer to contribute to the political bureau set up by the half-educated Nigerian dictator general Ibrahim Babangida in the mid-1980s, the Western Nigeria leader chief Obafemi Awolowo, stated that he could see no future unless the dialectics of the people changes. I had to search the meaning of the word "dialectics" in my dictionary. Indeed this right index finger, number two, trumps the thumb in the sense that you may vote in a supposedly democratic process with your thumb only to have a delusion of a government of the people. The half-education or non-education of the ruling elite and the non-stamping out of primitive customs of the people are part of today's schizophrenia of Africa.

3. **Economic philosophy:** Africa has none. In reality, economic and political philosophy go together, but the popular authors so far in this field of *Africa's problem with development* have not articulated any political and economic philosophical solutions unique to Africa's circumstances. Well, this is not surprising as it is academic custom for PhDs to load students and the world with academic analysis that can hardly ever come up with anything new. To this phenomenon the German philosopher Arthur Schopenhauer made a claim that all advances in philosophy, and perhaps in the real world of politics, are made outside academic walls, by activists perhaps. The fact that aid and other Western economic "help" to Africa has so far failed to work in Africa is a failure of academic economic philosophy that lacks genuine innovation. All talk and style, but no real substance in Africa's unique contexts. The reason may be because World Bank economists have simply ignored or not recognised the presence of the left hand and its fingers in African affairs and now that they attempt to unleash the right hand, they do so with a hand that has only the last 2 fingers! Looking back at the cold war era and 50 years of post-independence Africa, more madness is seen. I was surprised when an elderly Asian gentleman in the UK, but of Ugandan origin told me that *"Idi-Amin was a good man."* I thought Idi-Amin epitomised African psychopathic corruption and incompetence. This elderly Asian gentleman went on to explain to

me how an ordinary African was elevated by the ex-colonial masters to do their bidding, but the whole (mad) process went out of hand as part of the hot cold war in Africa. No better description of madness taking over normality is offered by the meaning of the name Mobutu Sese Seko Nkuku Ngbendu wa Za Banga. The bearer of this name with the help of the supposedly "ex-colonial masters" literally took the people's wealth for himself as there was no real "country," but a massive real estate, 70 times the size of the colonial master's own landmass. What economic philosophy were the backers of Mobutu applying at the time they put him there? Why blame the man who found himself in charge of another person's real estate? If the cold war was just about communism versus capitalism, not much blood should have been shed in Africa. The USSR should have given money to the state (which they did) and the West should have given money to the people (which they did not) and Africa would have been better as a result. Instead the imperialist philosophy and agendas of both the East and the West prevented the application of any genuine economic philosophy and the reality became a war of getting rid of the other's stooge. Capital and private wealth must belong to the people and the state must be the servant of the people with regard to this end, according to capitalism, I thought. In the midst of different versions of communism, I thought it basically stated that capital, wealth and production capacity must be owned collectively by the state. It is therefore my opinion that pure communism is unrealistic and unnatural. Nonetheless it must not be confused with socialism and our biological state of being inter-dependent and, therefore by default social animals that must reward the individuals who contribute most to the collective. So how does this biological and economic philosophy apply in Africa today? Far from it, nepotism, despotism and psychopathic corruption has made the most naturally economically productive individuals irrelevant in African politics! These individuals have emigrated and continue to do so, leaving the continent to remain more of the same – uneducated, corrupt and psychopathic. Any economic growth in such an environment can only be temporary, another false start and a waste of resources unless fingers number 1 and 2 are addressed and so far only a pan-African superstate seems to offer the platform to do so. Therefore any viable economic philosophy for Africa must incorporate fingers number 1 and 2 of the right hand.

4. **Institutions:** All over the world, various institutions serve as the unseen abstract, but highly effective hands of the state. What if the state is not real, but a sham? The government, the judiciary, the legislature, the press, the banking and monetary system, the educational institutions, etc., may be occupied by real people, but the outcome is hardly the objectives of a true state. It is of course easy to set up institutions in sham states, but what must happen in such scenarios is a primary school question and answer session - a joke! I remember in 1980 how embarrassed I was as an 8 year-old child, when a team of Nigerian athletes and officials were sent to the Moscow Olympic

Games. Nigeria went with the world's largest number of officials and came back with no medal! One official air-freighted a car on his way back. The point of citing this event is to show how the sporting institution of Nigeria was simply used by government officials for their own economic and frivolous ends. In other words, because there is no real country, those who happen to find themselves in government and all its institutions, use such institutions to further their individual objectives. Despite the 1980 embarrassment, Nigeria is still notorious for sending unnecessarily huge delegations to foreign events where most of the attendees do absolutely nothing for the country. We can extend this scenario to all the institutions of the country and see why they just don't work. I hear academics and all the gurus of international development trying to "strengthen" these institutions. Hmm, how naive! How possible is it to strengthen a psychiatric asylum run by schizophrenics? From the governments to the sporting institutions of some of these "countries," the effects of eight other fingers have created a beast that takes only a deep imagination and sense of history to see. Paul Collier noted that *"Even the appearance of modern government in these states is sometimes a facade, as if the leaders are reading from a script."* I smiled reading this from Collier's *The Bottom Billion.* Oh, another academic is only just now seeing the reality of what we have always seen and said, but no one heard because we truly have no voice in the global community bent on retaining the current colonial boundaries for the "states" of Africa. Why not call a sham a sham? We should not shy away from this fact or be frightened by it as it is not the same as taking responsibility for creating it; but its recognition will enable us address the reality of the issues emanating from it. Writing academically about the failings of a sham without calling it just that, is clear evidence of a lack of admission, or, genuinely not recognising it as a sham in the first place. No state should be regarded as a "failed state" when it was never a true state in the first place. There is no mystery here; the emergence of corrupt, incompetent and impotent judges, judiciary, legislators, presidents, governors and other administrators as the human component of a lot of African institutions is completely expected. I will therefore not go on to highlight the shambolism of every institution built on fake (not failed) states. All I can say is that new institutions need to be built from scratch with the benefit of hindsight (the left hand) and foresight (the right hand) that we now have regarding the problems of Africa. No other proposition other than a pan-African superstate offers a better opportunity to do this.

5. **Planning:** As the last of the fingers and just as small and seemingly unnoticeable as the left little finger (see above), this right little finger probably explains everything! Without it, the creative human hands will be incomplete and ineffective. When the Berlin Conference of 1884 to 1885 was held, what was the vision of 1985? Neither I nor any other African was at that great planning conference, but I could imagine what the naive expectation of 100 years later was. It

36

couldn't have been far from seeing the African continent reflecting European history and culture like the Americas. This of course is not a bad thing at all as Europe now means the "heaven" that lots of Africans dream of and choose to risk everything to emigrate to. Even in this letter, I dream of "SAAs" in Africa (mini-Utopias) with standards of governance and infrastructure no different from those of Western Europe. But all these are beside the point, and the issue now is what the plan for Africa is for the next 100 years. The planlessness in Africa post-independence is now easily understood in the context of the shambolism of most of her constituent states. Virtually all the drivers of the train (the state) are more concerned about remaining as the driver and enjoying the ride than they are about any destination that the train may be carrying its passengers to. Again, there can be no surprise here at all given the effects of all the other 9 fingers. O Barack, I cannot draw up a blueprint for how we can get to an Africa of our dreams in this letter, but I am sure we can do so if you use your position as the 44th president of The United States of America to influence America's foreign policy on Africa. I have offered the authentic voice of Africa and I propose that we must converge again in Berlin (symbolically) to plan the cure of Africa's schizophrenia.

Evaluating the 10 fingers

We must not at all give the impression that colonialism or European contact with Africa was completely bad or "evil", and that it is the main or only cause of Africa's woes of today. The slave trade probably did most of the damage in terms of altering the natural distribution of personality and other genetic traits of the indigenous population (unnatural selection), favouring the psychopath in the process. This is difficult to prove as are other mind entities, but others have written about this and I will not go into details here.

The scramble for Africa was probably a European mistake in hindsight. Left finger number 1 was, and remains the central evil in Africa till today and probably into the distant future as well. If not, why do most African politicians become politicians primarily for the sake of enriching themselves, despite knowing that they are incompetent, and sometimes too uneducated to occupy public office? O Barack, there is so much wickedness in Africa by Africans on Africans, to a point where the average African for now can only trust the outsider for genuine help even though the so-called evil of colonialism continues to be bandied about. Oh no, we would rather gamble with a stranger than work with our known enemies. Why do you think we keep our money – stolen and/or legitimately acquired – outside of Africa? In our hearts, we would rather trust our adopted mother (Europe) than adopted siblings (fellow "states"). As far as I am aware, colonialism actively helped to significantly reduce (but did not completely abolish) slavery in Africa. Pure slavery continues in Africa till today (2011)! But what would have happened to the continent of Africa had there been no European colonization or Berlin Conference between 1884 -1885?

The answer a medical student offered a long time ago was *"Islam would have spread southwards to the entire continent. For that alone we need to thank the colonial masters."* This is clearly a reflection of the bias that European colonisation brought in, but he probably should have said thank you for reducing (but not abolishing) the extremely wicked and superstitious practices of juju worshipers south of the Sahara. The spread of Islam in Africa was in itself a form of colonialism, as would any spread of religion with theocracy as the highly effective political ideology and a religious text as a quasi-constitution. It is interesting to note that Lord Frederick Lugard, the first Governor General of Nigeria did much to stop slavery in Africa. It is also interesting to note that I am only one generation from the generation that witnessed slavery and the killing of twins in the coast of West Africa. My mother grew up with some slaves of her great grandmother and I had two aunts who were killed as infants because they were born as twins. Today, I have twin sisters, something that my father was deprived of by his "traditions".

The question above takes us to another question. What if the Arabs and Europeans never got into North Africa thousands of years ago? Or indeed, what would have become of mankind had Homo sapiens and Neanderthals not crossed the Mediterranean ocean and the Sinai? Well, natural social evolution would probably have led to some form of theocracy or Han-like dynasty to dominate and populate the continent like it seems to have happened in China. Anyway, here we are with a contiguous land mass with possibly 2000 spoken languages and a billion people with a billion problems. What are we to do? In this modern time of universal human rights and values, how excellent and rewarding would it be to rebuild a whole continent from scratch with these values? How excellent and rewarding would it be to use the glory of our humanity combined with the magic of creativity and technology to build a new Africa? For the diversity of Africa can be made whole by universal human values – from fairness to compassion and from government of the people to government by the people for the people – and not the sham democracies that dots most of Africa.

That the problem of Africa is fundamentally political and therefore mind-related by default is no news, but I probably only have a say with regard to the mind. African economic problems are indirectly political, taking us to where we started – a mind-related problem. Erroneous scientific data and racist views had in the past implied that black Africans had a different brain and intelligence from other humans and that dark skin or melanin boosts libido. Some of these scientists tell us the truth about atoms, molecules and forces only to mislead us when it comes to human beings and their minds. In other words, they have the left hand of truth and the right hand of falsehood. Sometimes, it is difficult to differentiate one from the other. At this point it is worth remembering the statements of the very scientific and famous Nobel Prize-winning Professor James Watson, who helped discover the structure of DNA . . .

"[I am] inherently gloomy about the prospect of Africa [because] all our social policies are based on the fact that their intelligence is the same as ours—whereas all the testing says not really."

Most people now deal with the issue of racism with their hearts more than their heads, which is a good thing, but it is important to briefly re-clarify the true scientific position. It is a grave mistake to take association as the same as causation! Anything can be associated with dark skin, but both biological mechanism and history or "temporal sequence" are required to suggest a cause. Some racist scientists who scream about the infallibility of Darwinian evolution are quick to forget history (natural or unnatural) and the environment – the very ingredients for evolution, as they go about looking for delusional genes that they have erroneously assumed must make people mad or intelligent. The "genes" that are found more in psychiatric patients are also found in normal people, and the bulk of psychiatric patients have normal genes and brains. What does this tell us? Our theory of causation is faulty. We underestimate the manifestation of perceived abnormality as the result of human activities and constructs, as it is easier to blame nature. *"That's how you are,"* says the learned but misleading scientist. *"No, that's how I was made,"* I respond and add *"Indeed you don't know me, or do you? So*

40

how can you know how I am if you don't really know me? You are only just now hearing my authentic voice, silenced for half a millennium."

This is not about hiding under the umbrella of victimhood as politics follow the pattern of human social interaction, which itself is dependent on the human mind and brain. I will state that there are fundamental differences between the mind and the brain. The brain is the direct product of biology (physical reality and evolution), whilst the individual mind and "intelligence" are the abstract reflections of the individual's environment and developmental history, using the brain as an instrument or computer. There is no evidence that "processors" in the brain differ from one human race to another, and a significant difference is biologically implausible given that all humans are 99.5% identical DNA sequence-wise. In other words, the computer software (programs and memory as a whole) is quite distinct from the computer, even though one implies the existence of the other. We can speculate on "genetic pre-installation of programs in the brain and ancestral memories," considering the possibility of altered distribution of personality traits due to 400 years slavery, but ultimately, mind is memory and memory is mind. The "African mind" and the continent's current state is a reflection of her history very much like any individual human mind, disordered or otherwise is a reflection of individual history.

If we could homogenise the human social environment in one generation, we should expect to cancel out all racial and ethnic differences in mind-related measures. Stretching this metaphorically, I am tempted to conclude that ***the "African mind" is about the developmental history of both the African as an individual and the continent as a whole***. With all the pre-colonial, colonial and neo-colonial (mostly junk) memory occupying vital proximal disc space, in the form of corrupted colonial programs or "Apps", cookies and protocols what else, but the current state (schizophrenia) of Africa is expected? Those that are ignorant of Africa's history are eager to attempt

41

to re-write or overwrite on this disc with little free space. The solution is simple; the existing junk memory must be "maximally compressed" in such a manner that it does not affect thought processing (politics) anymore. This is the exact solution to the intractable psychological problem of personality disorders that result from childhood abuse, which science and psychologist cannot solve, because we do not know yet how to artificially compress thoughts.

There is however good news for Africa since Africa may have a mind, but is not a human being. The natural way for Africa to "maximally compress" her junk memory and apps is to get the AU big, strong and heavy enough to compress the arms of sham states and governments out of existence (relevance) to enable true ones (new apps) to grow and deliver the required functionalities – vision, competence and meritocracy. Achebe is right concerning the story (history) of the African peoples ...and the half a millennium of rain beating us. After 400 or 500 years, the sunshine must return to Africa. Where I come in once again as a psychiatrist is that I can easily point out that the brain does not have to be damaged for mental illness and/or other developmental disorders to occur. Indeed, although the disease, schizophrenia (the so-called "split mind") is frequently seen as a purely biological or brain problem, rarely (but understandably), do we find any physical abnormality in the individual brain, and when one is found, it is always non-specific and found in other individuals with other diseases or even without any obvious disease. It is a software problem, unknown to the "biological psychiatrist" who has no clue about the programming language of the mind. Once again, if we stretch this understanding metaphorically into the problem of Africa, we will all agree that virtually all the identifiable problems in Africa such as wickedness, corruption, ethnic/sectarian strife, self-serving leaders, etc., are not at all unique to Africa. Indeed, the events in Europe (the former Yugoslavia) less than 20 years ago, supports this position, although they are hardly explained by other people using psychiatric understandings/analogy. What is unique about the problem of Africa is her history – not the people! Picking on the history of Africa, it can be seen how the foundations of various African "countries" meant that what we are seeing today is completely expected and in line with their foundations. Martin Meredith quoted Ferhat Abbas's 1936 statement as follows:

"If I had discovered an Algerian nation, I would be a nationalist and I would not blush for it as though it were a crime. Men who die for a patriotic ideal are daily honoured and regarded. My life is worth no more than theirs. Yet I will not die for the Algerian homeland, because such a homeland does not exist. I have not found it. I have questioned history, I have asked the living and the dead, I have visited cemeteries: no one told me of it . . . One does not build on the wind."

Martin Meredith went ahead to quote Abubakar Tafawa Balewa and Obafemi Awolowo, two prominent pre- and post-independence "Nigerians".

". . . Nigerian unity is only a British intention" Said the one and *"There are no "Nigerians" in the same sense as there are "English", Welsh", or "French"* said the other.

Nonetheless, despite their observations no one took note of Ferhat Abbas's 1936 statement that " . . . One does not build on the wind," and a mere geographical expression (to quote Obafemi Awolowo) called Nigeria that officially came into existence as a geo-political entity in 1914, with the long term vision to be part of an empire was built upon. In just less than 50 years into the building project (1960), the original purpose and vision was abandoned and "independence" was offered to over 250 small nations (ethnic groups) that had been forcibly bound by their erstwhile colonial masters. Naturally, with the unnoticed building on the wind, the tendency was that individuals and individual ethnic groups – the real political entities – would seek self-determination without a specific new vision beyond "survival first" as there was hardly a new and true common aspiration that the collective had after the colonial masters handed over. Besides, prior to colonisation, these groups had political and religious systems in place and

43

these continued with a blend of what colonisation had brought in. It was this mix of pre-colonial tribal, political and religious agendas and post-colonial survival goals mixed with neo-colonisation – which included despots re-colonising the people and the cold war in Africa – that formed the faulty foundations of a lot of the newly "independent" schizophrenic African "countries." Indeed the civil wars in Africa were highly predictable in retrospect and the one that resulted in the brutal Nigeria civil war (1967 -1970) was the direct result of attempted self-determination by the Igbos gone awry.

When I make the statement "I am not really a Nigerian, but an Itsekiri and an African," even supposedly educated but in reality ignorant "Nigerians" fail to see the significance of such a truthful statement, and some genuinely talk about a "de-tribalised Nigeria," which would have been a good thing, if it had deep enough roots. "You mentally unemancipated slave, it is enough that you answer your master's name for you, but you should at least know who you really are!" I have said angrily in debates. So what can one expect of people in Europe and America who say "Africa is a very big country"? Ignorance of most things about Africa including her history and the true identities of the peoples of Africa is internally and externally pervasive! I cannot reasonably expect anyone living outside Nigeria to know about the Itsekiri people as they know about the Welsh.

Self-determination remains pivotal to both individual and state development, but how do we facilitate it without conflicts? Are there factors hindering the self-determination of individuals and states in Africa? The answer is YES in so many ways! For example, if Africa had the appropriate environment for her own professionals, we will not have rumours of over 20,000 Nigerian doctors and 200,000 African scientists allegedly in the USA and outside of Africa when at one stage there were only 20 doctors in the whole of one African country – Liberia. There are no reliable statistics in most parts of Africa and about Africans, but there is no doubt that there are millions of Africans abroad simply going after

44

their individual self-determination in more enabling environments - outside Africa. How come a lot of African "countries" have disabling social or political environments to their own people? I will come to this point later as I am one of the estimated 5000 Nigerian doctors in the UK alone. As I write this letter, my former schoolmates (doctors) are on strike in various parts of Nigeria over remuneration, as "legislators" pay themselves scandalous amounts of money ($1 million plus bribes) and ultimately 25% of the federal recurrent expenditure! O Barack, imagine if the U.S senate and House of Representative consumed 25% of the U.S federal budget. Why a Nigerian psychiatrist writing to the president of the USA makes sense after all, will become apparent when we see once again that the "disabling environment" in Africa is not the physical environment but the minds of the people who hold power and authority over others' wish for self-determination. Self-determination may continue to go awry so long as the faulty foundations and environments are built on. For example Al-Shabaab's attempt to rule Somalia is part of self-determination that will continue to go awry . . . just like other attempts, such as the botched democratization in Algeria in 1991, caused by the imminent emergence of Islamic Salvation Front as the democratically elected government of Algeria, based on religious extremism. So clearly, Africa's history has showed that the government of the people, by the people may produce an unwise government. This is basically related to faulty foundations as it is elsewhere in the world, but more so in Africa. This is why I believe Africa must be "born again" by rebuilding continental social structures (mind-related environments) without the current faulty foundations of its dysfunctional colonial, and neo-colonial past, using the benefit of both hind- and foresights.

I am an African and belong to the Itsekiri tribe. These are my natural identities, but it is interesting to note that with my grandfather being made a Nigerian in 1914, I was offered Nigerian citizenship comparable to the British citizenship I received in 2006 with a deep sense of gratitude for the kindness of the British people and the Queen of England. Today, I am officially an individual of dual nationality: "British - Black African" is what I fill in forms for "equal opportunities". When will Africa get here? This is the identity story of millions of people of African descent and in this identity are the wet clothes of the rain that we have endured for hundreds of years. Poverty, hunger, poor economic growth and development despite Africa's wealth and the advancement of mankind in the 21st century can only be a mind-related problem; the schizophrenia of a continent where the presence of wickedness, corruption and greed meant that only a few that remained on the soil of Africa managed to attain a decent standard of life when compared to the experience of western Europe and the United States.

From time to time we see African "patriots" and despots on television talking about the unity of their "countries" and they are quick to spew out statements against "neo-colonialism" whilst benefiting from the spoils of colonialism (mere geographical expressions with huge bank accounts meant for countries run by a few indigenous families and cabals). This is an act of wickedness and not ignorance, for such individuals are quick to jump back to their tribal, sectarian or religious roots in times of trouble because they were never interested in true federalism in the first place. O Barack, your sister Auma was right; that some people took over the colonial master's place, but simply committed worse exploitation and wickedness to the people. You are familiar with this story for your father suffered the consequences.

True federalism in Africa can only be offered by a pan-African superstate – big enough to be above racism and tribalism, strong enough to eliminate the demon of psychopathic corruption and self-serving rulers and united in spirit, truth and purpose to ensure economic growth for the people.

The wickedness in Africa is from within and from without; but the history of Africa is clear in showing that it was the external wickedness that fed the internal one, just as the external

46

corruption continues to feed the internal one till date; the best U.S - related one being between Halliburton and Nigerian "government" officials. If there are no dodgy "out of court settlements," no safe Swiss banks for stolen African monies, and no unsupervised Oil companies, perhaps Africa's resources and cash would be invested in Africa. If there are no external supporters of despots, perhaps genuine democracy will flourish in all of Africa.

Africa's psychopathic corruption
No discussion about the problems of Africa will be complete or even make headway without an understanding of its unique form of corruption. From time to time, we hear frank and very enlightened pundits admitting that "corruption is everywhere" and so in Africa, it is neither a unique problem, not the main cause of the continent's underdevelopment. This view, sadly, is uninformed and drastically underestimates the devastating effects of Africa's brand of corruption because no one has explained that Africa has a unique form of corruption - psychopathic corruption. African psychopathic corruption is indeed unique because it simply doesn't care and derives pleasure in seeing people suffer . . . and in extreme cases involves satanic ritual murders in the process of integrating juju worshipers into government. Surely, this kind of corruption is not the same as simple bribes and kickbacks in the United States for example, and must be uniquely devastating and unbelievable in the 21st century, except that it is true at least in Nigeria. No economic policy can ever work with this pre-historic kind of corruption. All growth will be temporary.
Why would uneducated, conspicuously incompetent, and known and convicted criminals seek to occupy public office? Why, in any country would the majority of politicians seek public office and political power with the primary intention of self-enrichment and secondary intention of fraudulent leadership? Why would professors and so-called intellectuals gladly put themselves at the disposal of criminals? Why would

47

legislators pay themselves millions of dollars and seize 25% of the federal budget for themselves, as the citizens of the country starve and infrastructure decay? Simple answer; the environment of widespread psychopathic corruption allows it. Only a united Africa carries any hope of changing this environment and to create a disincentive for incompetent people to smell public office. The effect of the slave trade leaving sub-Saharan Africa with psychopaths has to be true; otherwise it becomes easier to blame Africa's unique corruption on genetic or innate factors such as intelligence that are unique to dark-skinned individuals. Kind and caring bookworms like my father and I don't (actually couldn't) generally do well financially and politically in Africa, but my less caring and psychopathic brother, uncle and cousins do (did). It is my opinion that to survive in the local environment (of inter- and intra-tribal wars) that supported the slave trade for 400 years, you had to be a psychopath . . . who simply don't (can't) care and must have the demise, oppression, subjugation, captivity, imprisonment and sale of your brother to survive! 400 years may not be too short in terms of mind and evolutionary adaptation to the environment and we may have taken a backward or regressive evolutionary step that required the awakening of previously silent genes or ancestral memories; and a metaphorical return to the Garden of Eden and a new dialogue with Satan.

Psychopathy . . . widespread psychopathy is probably the single most important factor that explains the persistence of Africa's underdevelopment. Psychopaths are not compassionate and this explains why most "leaders" of Africa are not just self-serving, but they seem not to notice the sufferings around them because they don't really (and by nature, cannot) care and damn the consequences of their actions on others. Surely, the sheer scale of thieving in Nigeria (an estimated 80% of government revenue) and the hidden wealth and callousness of African "leaders" such as Equatorial Guinea's Obiang (sadly, the chairperson of the current infantile AU as I write you this letter), in the midst of dire poverty of their people are proofs that they must be psychopaths. It is my deep desire that academics who have talked about "Hubris syndrome" in western politicians will see the validity of psychopathic corruption as possibly the single virus that cascades the intractable developmental disorder of Africa. Indeed the metaphorical return to the Garden of Eden and a new dialogue with Satan in Africa becomes concrete when we consider the fact that a lot of African corruption is actually linked to juju worship and high political office holders actually do participate in satanic rituals as a pre-condition for being offered office or joining an "elite" group.

To conclude this chapter about the problem of Africa, I have to say that my views are not new and I am not alone. I have deliberately not mentioned others who have more recently been pushing for a United States of Africa such as Muammar Gaddafi until now. Gaddafi, sadly and despite his vocal pan-Africanist position, was part of the sham leadership and schizophrenia of Africa. I am genuine (as a messenger) and along with the African blogosphere, united in the demand for authenticity in African affairs:
   "What makes decolonization and Independence failures makes Self Determination successful. Self Determination starts with the premise that a people / group have original inalienable rights of Sovereignty and independence and should have control over their destiny and resources: their nationhood, dignity and humanity ought to be recognized and respected. Self Determination is people-centered; and in so far as the "State" is concerned, Self Determination avers and insists that the right of the people takes precedence over the State—naturally because it is in fact the people who make the State; it should not be the other way around."
- Oguchi Nkwocha, MD, Nwa Biafra. A "Biafran Citizen" on "Why Decolonization And Independence Don't Work Where Self Determination Would" (March 3, 2011 on www.saharareporters.com)

In all these, it is worth repeating that it is not an exaggeration to state that all arms of government in most "states" of Africa (with the most populous "state" in Africa – Nigeria - as the best example) are a complete sham; for the essence of a sham is in its looking like the real thing! The more it looks like the real thing, the more it is a sham; but in the end, a sham is a sham.

Chapter 3

The Solution: A True African Union

U.S looking for New Course in Africa, says Clinton.
Charting a new course for sustainable U.S. engagement with
Africa is vital, Secretary Hillary Rodham Clinton tells U.S.
envoys at the African Chiefs of Mission Conference. "What
happens in Africa has a very direct and growing impact on
what happens in Europe and what happens in the United
States." ...

- www.america.gov (Susan Domowitz, staff writer)

There is only one very clear path for the U.S to follow and it is
to support a true African Union and do so with passion and
commitment. All "Africans" uniting means the whole of
mankind uniting to accelerate the political and socio-economic
integration of the cradle of civilization – the continent of
Africa; to promote and defend African common positions on
issues of interest to the continent and its peoples; to achieve
peace and security in Africa; and to promote democratic
institutions, good governance and human rights - the very aims
and objectives of the African Union as it stands today.
The beauty of an idea is not just in its ability to capture a story
in an instant, but in its ability to reduce a mountain to a stone.
Taking on the problems of a continent with roughly 30 million
square kilometres in size and a billion people is more than
climbing a mountain. It needs spiritual and divine intervention.
However, this mountain has been reduced to a stone in this
letter and the divine intervention is at hand! Now what shall
we do with the stone O Barack? We are divinely guided in the
bible which states that the stone must be thrown at the feet of

the mighty statue of king Nebuchadnezzar (Daniel chapter 2:31-35 – The Bible):

Your Majesty looked, and there before you stood a large statue—an enormous, dazzling statue, awesome in appearance. [32] The head of the statue was made of pure gold, its chest and arms of silver, its belly and thighs of bronze, [33] its legs of iron, its feet partly of iron and partly of baked clay. [34] While you were watching, a rock was cut out, but not by human hands. It struck the statue on its feet of iron and clay and smashed them. [35] Then the iron, the clay, the bronze, the silver and the gold were all broken to pieces and became like chaff on a threshing floor in the summer. The wind swept them away without leaving a trace. But the rock that struck the statue became a huge mountain and filled the whole earth.

O dear Barack . . . you are familiar with the bible . . . a book that does not mean what is written in it, but means much more! Those ignorant of things spiritual will be lost at this point, but the mountain of the reality of administering a continent and a billion people is not new; for China and India are there to learn from. My role as a messenger is simply to advise you to throw this stone (the rock cut out of a mountain, but not by human hands - Daniel 2:45) . . . and as has happened before, Goliath will be brought down with a stone and Daniel's prophesy will come to pass . . . and the rest, as they say will become history. Technocrats, architects, Pan-African enthusiasts, friends of Africa, spiritual Africans (of no race), entrepreneurs and all kinds of professionals are waiting to sort out the details of this stone. The destination is clear: a truly politically united Africa built on fundamental and universal positive human values. The only thing that may hinder the throwing of this stone is the cry of those who are benefiting from the status quo. They will cry the wolf of neo-colonialism whilst at the same time benefiting from the remnants of the spoils of colonialism ("real estate states" with huge bank accounts and quasi-slave workers) and neo-colonialism (mineral exploiting companies, middlemen posing as government and the cold war): O Barack, do not listen to them, for a true pan-African superstate means the end of neo-colonialism!

Daniel 2:44- 45: *"In the time of those kings, the God of heaven will set up a kingdom that will never be destroyed, nor will it be left to another people. It will crush all those kingdoms and bring them to an end, but it will itself endure forever. [45] This is the meaning of the vision of the rock cut out of a mountain, but not by human hands—a rock that broke the iron, the bronze, the clay, the silver and the gold to pieces.*

The AU as it is in 2011 and what should happen next

The concept of a United States of Africa is not new, and the fact that it has so far not been seriously considered is due to the power of incumbency. Why would any sitting despot such as Robert Mugabe or Obiang Nguema (sadly the current chairperson of the AU) agree to a vision that would mean his end? Without careful consideration, the idea of a Pan-African superstate is easily dismissed by the small-minded as an impractical imitation of the EU and even undesirable from Africa's unique socio-cultural standpoint. Yet, it is Africa that needs unity more than Europe as we cannot run away from the basic notion of *united we stand, divided we fall*: Africa remains the best place on earth to exploit people and their states because the people are divided. In the Savannahs of Africa, we see clearly how the lion preys more easily on the individual animal separated from the pack. China is now the new lion preying on separated African buffalos. So why can't Nigerians, needless to mention Africans as a whole, truly unite? Are we too fundamentally different and bigoted to ever unite for a common purpose (for example to prevent our collective exploitation)? My answer is NO! All of mankind can unite for a common purpose if the goal is shared and well defined. Perhaps as individuals, we find it hard to really appreciate and accept the value or indispensability of another person who is not very much like us. This is the weakness of the bigot and small-minded. There is no point in paying lip service to concepts such as *"there is strength in diversity"* when most of us do not really appreciate what the underlying strength of diversity really entails. If we did, then no group of persons in Nigeria would ever imagine killing youths whose stated purpose was to unite the country or burn people to death for whatever reason as we saw happen in Ivory Coast and Libya in 2011. This is evidence of Africa's deep-seated bigotry and ignorance of what diversity really entails. A shared purpose is the underlying ingredient that strengthens a diverse group of anything including humans in an ecosystem or machine components! The problem with Africans as a whole is that our (fake or basically incompetent) leaders and technocrats do not share our purpose. They have their own selfish agendas, like the imperialists did pre-independence or misunderstand the true sense of the word, diversity. If the technocrats who fly with our leaders to AU meetings understood the benefits of diversity, then a union government would have been in place by now. Agreed, leadership has been identified as a critical factor for Africa's current underdevelopment and I was made to believe that this was why you chose Ghana and not Nigeria for your first visit to sub-Saharan Africa. I read your speech to the Ghanaian parliament in full and you indirectly agreed that it was Africa's history that gave birth to rulers (non-leaders) as leaders, but that is still no excuse as Africa's future is up to Africans and we must stop blaming colonialism of the past for the problems of the present. I cannot challenge your position, but while conceding that leadership is the key to Africa's development, we Africans are placed in a precarious situation when we have leaders who do not have it within their intellectual capacity to have a true vision for diverse peoples. Worse still, is when such leaders do not truly represent their people's interests. You pointed a finger to Mugabe in your speech. This is a serious matter and it is clear that Africa has had illiterate and half-educated "leaders" who just cannot be expected to see beyond ethnic, tribal and other parochial agendas. If we had genuinely visionary leaders, then a Union

54

Government will be top of the AU's agenda at each annual meeting until such a meeting transforms itself into the Union Government's facilitation of an annual "grand joint congressional meeting" instead of the current annual heads of state jamboree. We cannot turn back the hands of time, but those Africans, especially technocrats, who now claim to be educated and enlightened enough to see the bigger picture and the strength in diversity, must now use their intellectual prowess and creativity to create a new future for Africa that specifically excludes our current psychopathically corrupt and usually incompetent "leaders" by building a pan-African superstate big and diverse enough to be above tribalism, and nepotism; strong enough to eliminate the demon of psychopathic corruption and self-serving rulers; sophisticated and intellectually challenging enough to exclude half-educated politicians from government and united in spirit, truth and purpose enough to actually work in practice to ensure economic growth for the people.

One look at how the existing AU is constituted at the moment shows a government in evolution. Indeed the debate at the July 2007 AU summit held in Ghana, focused on the creation of a Union Government and a United States of Africa. This is not surprising to those familiar with the history of modern Africa, as Kwame Nkrumah the first president of Ghana and others such as Patrice Lumumba and Jomo Kenyatta as far back as the 1940s saw the image of a truly united Africa just like Marcus Garvey saw in the 1920s. The creation of a union government has stalled, and the current AU "parliament" composed of 265 representatives from all 53 AU states is of course anything but a parliament. To begin with, the schizophrenia of the various African "states" and numerous delusions of the despots who claim to represent such states need to be cured. My belief expressed here may sound rather extreme and unfair to some, but the attitudes of the average African president suggests that he does not truly represent his people, but himself! This schizophrenia was demonstrated in the fact that the most vocal proponent of a pan-African superstate at the time I wrote the first draft of this letter was being bombed by Western powers to protect his people from him, and the chairperson of the AU at the same period, was arguably the worst dictator in Africa – worse than Mugabe! Therefore AU summits attended by unrepresentative leaders may always stop short of agreeing on laws and projects that will see genuine people-representation that would spell the end of most African "leaders." To prove my point further in the dynamic situation involving Libya, the AU was completely useless at the height of the conflict and when the rest of the world supported the people, the AU supported a dictator! This is why the creation of a union government by the AU has stalled. The cure for the schizophrenic illness is not to immediately abandon the current colonial boundaries (that will be a recipe for disaster), but to recognise at a continental level, all the political and tribal entities, no matter how small and innumerable they may be, in Africa prior to European colonisation. The predecessor to the AU, the Organisation of African Unity (OAU), proved itself for a long time between 1963 – 2002 to be not just impotent, but also as a club of dictators. The AU as it is at the moment is different from the OAU only in name and has proved itself useless in the arena of conflict resolution and the fight against corruption where we are still relying on our erstwhile colonial masters to tackle serious conflicts (more recently in Ivory Coast and Libya) and prosecute our thieves (James Ibori in London) and murderers (Charles Taylor at The Hague) in government. Events in the Ivory Coast, Sudan, Libya, Somalia, Zimbabwe, and virtually everywhere the AU is expected to be useful, demonstrates its impotence. Yet, it is a strong pan-African superstate with one army and a common market that will obviate the need for foreign military and economic intervention in African affairs. Yes, Africa needs only one professional 21st century army and not the useless armies across Africa that recurrently seize the (colonial-boundary) state in unnecessary coups, make themselves instruments of despots, kill their own people and rape their own women.

United we stand and divided we fall, needs no explanation as African peoples, not states, are weakened and left economically impotent at least in part, by remaining cut off from their natural parts – contiguous borders and natural markets! We all know why companies merge. It is for their mutual economic interests. The practical benefits of merging to companies such as cost savings and sharing of expertise are no different from those to states; but Africa's regional economic integration and their inefficiency reflects the incompetence of policy makers who simply copy others, but don't know why others have done what they did. The practicalities of uniting Africa's markets will not be as challenging as uniting its thousands of tribal nationalities. First uniting the 54 post-colonial "countries" will seem like the most practicable way to proceed, but if all the ethnic nationalities genuinely have a common aspiration (purpose) such as genuine economic advancement with no false starts, and not how to defeat a political rival, neighbouring tribe or region, then we will unite underneath our colonial boundaries – with strategic economic policies and accountability left to the continental government.

I know that most African rulers will not push for unity due to incompetence and lack of political will against their personal interests, but the people will, if the international community invests in the people and not their governments. Yes, it is the international community that will facilitate Africa's unity to obviate the need for the same international community to persistently drop by to resolve conflicts that can be linked to disunity in the first place. Libya's story is the proof. So how can we unite the people without uniting their governments? Simple! The international community must themselves first be united in retailoring their individual foreign policies for Africa to be centred on a demand for a truly united Africa in the form of a superstate. The people of Africa will naturally unite when there is free migration to prosperous places within the continent.

People tend to naturally unite for the sake of their own economic benefits which filter into the economy of the collective. Therefore, proposed Special Administrative Areas or Special Economic Zones with free migration based on manpower needs alone, will unite people from all over the continent. If these SAAs and SEZs are dotted across the continent and controlled by the new AU, then the people will unite without significant involvement of their government. The question left is how to ensure that these special areas or zones become prosperous. This is where the international community and aid providers come in and this will be explained in the later aspects of this chapter. The practical aspects of uniting Africa should begin by investing in the peoples of Africa. The continent's social order needs a complete overhaul where each African alive today needs to be allowed to speak in a referendum that is free and fair to decide whether or not he or she wants to be bound by a continental constitution which will be centred on the governing of their governments and the judging of the judiciaries of all existing states and tribes, based on universal positive human values and genuine implementation to the letter and in spirit.

This cannot be done with Africa's current institutions that have dug in, covertly or "mind-wise," to protect the interests of a few elite whose economic and political survival depends on the unfairness and injustices of the status quo. Politics, according to Will Durant, is not as one might suppose, the art and science of capturing and keeping office, but the study of ideal social organisation. Africa's current social organisation or politics is far from ideal for its unique circumstances and this explains all the continents problems. It needs re-engineering. Therefore, a true government for the whole continent naturally holds the sustainable solutions for the problems. This will immediately lead to a rebirth of the authentic African and enable delusions such as the "Nigerian" to be put in appropriate context. This context should be represented by a tribal congress as the house of parliament that decides finally on the future of all African peoples with the basic human aim of self-determination. With this congress, why would any tribe or people take up arms to fight against marginalisation and oppression by a neighbouring tribe or even a despot, when "big brother African tribal congress" will always be on your side - the side of peace and self-determination? This should be the house superior to the African senate made up of 200 seats (100 population-based seats, 54 country-based seats and 46 GDP and other important factor-based seats). The senate would of course legislate on all matters, but can have any of its laws overturned by the tribal house. The tribal house should also have the power to direct the executive on any continental issue. At this point the concept of a tribal house from a distance must once again look impracticable, until we genuinely realise that there is strength in diversity, not just as a cliché or food for lip service, and more so if the strength is built on authentic identities; first at the local "wards" or street level then onto towns, regions, countries and finally the continent. This of course, takes us to the issue of unreliable data and corrupted population figures for the sake of political manipulations: Pan-African institutions such as Office for Statistics, Census Commission, Continental Electoral Commission and Social Security will help transform local politics for good. If run properly these proposed continental institutions can turn data into lives saved and the people genuinely empowered (more on this later). The tribal parliament will be a wonderful opportunity to democratise existing African traditional institutions where if a dunce is the king, too bad for his followers. All that needs to be done is to copy the UK democracy by leaving hereditary monarchies as they are, but insist that they have largely traditional and ceremonial roles and that only an elected tribal prime minister can represent the people at the African Tribal House and the Federal Houses of Representatives in their existing colonial states. This will do the Swazi people a lot of good. Elections should be conducted by an African Continental Electoral Commission (ACEC). Undoubtedly, if an African Electoral Commission, free of the influence of despots conducts elections from the ward or street level to the continental level, using appropriate technology and centrally-secure data (population data matched to the electoral and social security registers), sham elections will be a thing of the past. We should also expect swift and credible judicial reviews if required, as well as immediate military intervention from our single army to kick out bad losers – the Ratsirakas and Gbagbos of Africa – by force. This takes us straight to the need to invest in (counting and accounting for) the people and not the existing states of Africa. The people's social security and not state security will be a good start for such an investment.

Investing genuinely in the people of Africa for the first time in history!

The first time the world was truly interested in the inhabitants of sub-Saharan Africa on a large scale was during the slave trade; to use the people outside the continent. Pre-slave trade interests in Africa were not on a large scale and the trade was insignificant. The next time of interest in the inhabitants of the continent on a large scale was to convert the people to labourers in their own lands, but to the benefit of others - colonialism! There have of course been various kinds of interests in Africa with little to do with the people; for example for the wildlife, the minerals, the forests, the deserts to test Atomic weapons, unfair trade, proxy wars, and so on. There has also been the occasional genuine curiosity about culture, interesting leaders and interesting people, but not on a large scale. What is now getting close to a large scale in terms of interests in people inhabiting Africa is in the area of charity and disease control. How sad! The people of Africa are now stereotyped with pictures of malnourished children, AIDS and war. Under such circumstances interests in the people for the sake of meeting their charitable needs is perfectly understandable. But this misses the true picture of the people – the history of a development disorder. **The only charity**

needed by the people is not strictly a charitable gesture, but it is about proactively preventing the people from being exploited by a new empire, kingdom (China or other so-called emerging markets) or despot (fake nationalist). Preventing further exploitation of Africa probably can only be done by truthfully ensuring that there is a strong United Nations Security Council resolution (O yes, this is a security issue!) that first of all guarantees the sovereignty of all authentic tribes and small nations of Africa, followed by each existing colonial state in Africa truthfully ensuring that there is genuine citizen rights through **counting and accounting for everyone,** by **offering the role of judge of the efficacy of their laws to the AU.** When the colonial state is the Judge of its own human rights enforcement, we get Libya's shambolism of being in the UN's Human Rights Council whilst killing its own people as a means of sustaining the rule of its despot. Who really cares about the common man in Africa? I have asked myself. Putting missionaries and self-sacrificing charity workers aside, the clear answer is no one! O yes, no one. For I have seen it in Egypt and in Nigeria and heard and read about it almost everywhere else in Africa where the government is basically incompetent or office-holders simply don't care – most of Africa. All the aid given to African "governments" should never have been given to them! It should have been given directly or indirectly to the ordinary people, individuals or companies whose directors could have been held personally responsible. Funding or supporting unrepresentative governments is the reason why aid has failed to make much of a difference to Africa.

The investment in the people of Africa must begin with gathering data, but exactly how many people to the last digit really live in the continent of Africa? How many "Nigerians" are there? No one really knows the answer as data from Africa is generally unreliable and frequently outright falsifications! No Nigerian census has been regarded as credible because of a perceived need to manipulate the figures for political and economic gains, but from estimates we know that roughly100 to 200 million people live in the geographical area called Nigeria. Should we start with an African continental census? Why not? But who will fund the census? This is where a challenge is thrown to all who intend to invest in Africa's future. This is also where creativity, entrepreneurialism and 21st century capitalism and technology can come in beautifully:

The proposed Continental Census as the hallmark of genuinely investing in the people of Africa on a large scale for the first time and rebuilding Africa's institutions.

Some have proposed strengthening existing African institutions as an essential way to foster economic growth. This is very true, as the AU is itself an existing institution. However, supposing some institutions you wish to strengthen had no real foundations, will you not be attempting to prop a skyscraper that was built from within 2 feet of earth? What if some of the institutions you wish to strengthen include shambolic parliaments with no real powers and corrupt or incompetent judges? Can we strengthen shams? NO! I say, and certainly not when the fundamental problem is one of the mind; with ignorance, dishonesty and psychopathy at the core. Woe unto those who attempt to change a nation without first changing the people! New and innovative institutions must be rebuilt from scratch, with an architecture specifically designed to be people-orientated, rigorous and transparent enough to keep incompetence and psychopathic corruption out of the way. The new AU offers a wonderful and exclusive opportunity for innovation. For Africa, only the AU can bring in, and dig deep the necessary foundations, if honest people, irrespective of nationality and governments, seize the initiative before unrepresentative "heads of states" gather and sabotage the appropriate people-based foundations of our proposed new AU.

Now, why count people simply for the sake of numbering them when you can use the process to do a lot more? Has anyone imagined the proposed African single currency being linked to a census? No, because it will only take the imagination of passionate dreamers and visionaries to do so. Now, if I am offered $100 to provide my biometric data after which I will be put in the African census register, offered a social security card, a visa credit card, a mobile phone SIM card, an African Continental Passport and a voter registration card, I certainly will take the offer - like most Africans home and abroad will . . . and we are all counted. Will it be too expensive, as to make it basically impossible? No, not if the spirit is to genuinely invest in the peoples of Africa; to count everyone, account for everyone and pay quasi-reparations for slavery! Poor data in Africa is the root of planlessness and state services failures in Africa. Money spent in this area of sophisticated population and personal data gathering if well spent, will have an impact like never before and be positively judged by history. Well, $100 per person without the overhead cost of the whole process, translates into $100 billion dollars. What if it is locked in the new common currency? Who will use it? Where will they use it? Who will begin to accept the "Frika" (not the "Afro" which is too much of an imitation of the Euro as already proposed)? At this point, bankers whom "I hear" create money out of thin air may begin to see how they can fund our continental census and make some very ethical profit for themselves in the process. I will leave the issue of the common single African currency to the imagination of bankers for now and move on to the issue of accounting for everyone with the social security card.

I am unfamiliar with concepts of social security in Africa – families are natural social security to each other – but I know that technology-wise, Africans have no problems using smart devices. Now with the new ASSC (African Social Security Card) no one will ever need to go to feeding camps. Why? You may ask: Because it is a credit card! No need for aid to be given to sham governments anymore when the people can have the cash shared and dispensed electronically! All people need do is go to the shop that accepts the card, and since the card contains dollars, food from all parts of the earth will find their way to where the card is. There will be no need for complex and expensive charity operations, as capitalism will take its natural course. Interestingly, but sadly before I could get my thoughts and suggestions out to the public, the East Africa famine had begun and the 1980s tragic sight of starvation and "walking skeletons" re-emerged as a disgraceful reality of Africa in the 21st century. The feeding camps returned and the foreign, usually Western aid workers came to Africa's rescue. O, I wish the ASSC was already in place. Part of the 60 – 80% of aid money that goes into the administration of the aid itself, would have been channelled into the ASSC.

Even individual philanthropy could use this technology: A personal donation from an individual anywhere in the world could go directly to an individual ASSC. It will be no different from the "sponsoring a child" programme that a lot of charities do, but more direct and cost-effective. It will deprive a lot of charity workers or their current administrative duties, but will create new and better jobs for the same charity workers and importantly, for Africans as well.

Every child at birth should be coded from hospital or at the registry. Maternity and hospital licensing will require coding technology. Children who attend school will have ASSC school cards at registration and uniforms with bar coding thereafter, which will automatically be scanned to register attendance. Such a card for African children will get most of them to take school more seriously. How nice will it be to deduct cash from these school cards for bad behaviour and top up the cards with cash for good behaviour and academic achievements? I would have made my parents some money in my time . . . if ASSC existed between 1976 and 1987. This is how in the 21st century Africa must account for her new generation. I was surprised, shocked with a sense of validation, to find out that thoughts that I had arrived at from my own meditations are not at all new. Indeed I have just described another version of "conditional cash transfer" and its immense benefits to the people. *The scheme has met with resounding success in developing countries, so why has this type of programme not been rolled out aggressively across Africa?* This critical question was posed by Dambisa Moyo. Did someone see the vanishing away of sham elections in Africa with the advent of the ASSC? Politically conscious Nigerians will, as Nigeria recently conducted one of the most expensive voter registration exercises in the world so far - about $0.6 billion - to register about 70 million people and still could not come up with a credible election. I was not registered as the existing Nigerian government could not be bothered with those of us living abroad. With biometric data collected for multiple and long term purposes such as birth and death registrations, social security, travel documentation or identification, manipulation specifically of electoral registers will be impossible and updates will be pretty simple, not requiring a specific period prior to elections. Indeed, this whole process can begin tomorrow if all African Governments consent to the modernisation of all existing local registry offices. It was rather unintelligent for Nigeria to waste $0.6 billion on a voter's registration exercise that allegedly involved the registration of non-Nigerians and under-aged persons for the purpose of rigging the election. We may as well register all Africans. Besides, with SMS technology linked to ASSC and registered voters by default, we could survey the political views and likely voting patterns prior to an election. Indeed, there will be no need for a Gallup poll as the SMS-linked ASSC can deliver very reliable data if holders are incentivised to text. Aha! Did I hear that Vodafone may be interested in our census? Which mobile phone company wants to have a customer from birth and for life? Do you want the African to have cash in his pocket before you give him a SIM card or give him the SIM card and expect him to need to make a call later? Again, as with the bankers, I'll leave it to the imaginations of those who know their markets.

It is worth noting that sham governments do have departments of planning and statistics. However, what can we expect? The planlessness in Nigeria for example was demonstrated by the rising population and rising number of cars over a 20 year period (1980 -2000) without anyone taking notice only for fuel scarcity to become the norm in a country that exports the raw material for petroleum products. This is not surprising when successive drivers of a car are more concerned about remaining as the driver than the destination of the car. This is the journey of Africa's post-independence history so far; with incompetent drivers holding on to the steering wheel of our car. No data, no statistics. Poor statistics means poor planning. No statistics means building on the wind – the faulty foundations of most African states with sham governments. Statistics aside, the human beings in Africa are real and have real human issues as they do their best to try to survive and maintain order. O Barack, who really cares about these people? Those who wield power simply sit on their gains and steal as much as they can. Who will plan for the people when they have no real governments? It is only by investing in the people first and foremost, that the people can then plan for themselves and their legitimate and elected governments. Thereafter, the truly representative governments can plan the management of the natural resources and economy of the continent for the benefit of the human inhabitants and the world at large.

There is a population explosion going on in Africa. Has anyone taken note? Reports indicate that sub-Saharan Africa has the world's most youthful population and it is projected to stay that way for decades. The African continent is expected to have 349 million youths and 29 per cent of the world's total population come 2050. Imagine everyone in the USA aged between 15 and 24.Who is planning for all these youths in these geographical delineations with sham governments?

66

Would it not be useful to have the ASSC as a women empowering and educational tool that would enhance family planning? As an indirect fertility control tool, it will be controversial but feasible; two children per woman after which all social services support is stopped. Compulsory health and family planning education should follow the first child, and compulsory sterilisation should be offered in exchange for the social support for the 3rd child.

With the common people of Africa as the first focus of thought and investments, what should come next?

The political unification of Africa will begin to happen naturally as pan-African projects begin to happen. In other words, if a process of capitalising the AU and carrying out a continental census begins, so will the political unification. Similarly, the planning and execution of other trans-continental projects such as trans-continental roads, rail, power plants and "continental cities" under the supervision of the true AU can only cement the unification further.

If the AU is imagined not as a government initially, but as a multinational company or "PLC" set up to invest in the people, it will be easy to see how practicable the unification projects will turn out. After all, we cannot forget the colonial history and role of companies such as the Royal Niger Company. "Capitalising" the AU will not threaten any existing despot, but help the people who are suffering under him. Under these proposals, unless the despot uses restriction of the movement of people and wickedness as bargaining tools I cannot see why he will oppose continental development projects in "his" territory. For example, if the AU proposes to build a Continental city along the Zimbabwe-South Africa border (an area of so much tears and blood), I cannot see why

Robert Mugabe would object. It would not take much from him, but the project will offer his people refuge and a place to rebuild the lives he ruined. I will come back to the very important issue of continental cities, but I will state at this point that I do not think starting a city is difficult if there is collective will. If there is fertile land, water, a rumour of the presence of gold in the land, a self-sustaining city will spring up! That is the work of the human mind. The "gold" in any land we choose will be AU and aid or "quasi-reparations money to share" – this should get emigration-prone West Africans scampering to these new cities and Europe (especially Italy's Lampedusa) may get some respite as a result. Such cities will be SARs or SAAs (Special Administrative Regions or Special Administrative Arrangements). If mighty China inadvertently benefitted massively from SARs and SEZs, Africa too can seize such benefits. If mighty China can have "one country, two systems," why should any African country claim a threat to sovereignty or neo-colonialism with our economically potent concept of SAAs? Most Africans may not want to openly admit it (although some Nigerians agree); that South Africa as the richest country in Africa today, despite its dark history, owes its success to being a form of SAR within the African continent!

The most important question at this stage is where will the start-up capital for this mega company (capitalised AU) come from? As with any start-up, it is about value creation, people being interested in the created "valuables," credit, buying and selling all together at the same time. Africa through the AU certainly has a lot to buy and sell, but who is creating the value in the minds of people and who is genuinely interested? Value and credit are human mind-related entities and if the AU becomes a genuine representative and instrument of the common man of Africa, then the middlemen (corrupt so-called leaders) who are currently exploiting the people will lose their "jobs." Let Us imagine that henceforth all foreign aid to Africa and charitable activities must be through the AU. Straightaway, the company has $50 billion of capital coming in the form of grants every year. Well, this will mean all those "technical assistance" and cash that never physically reached the continent in the past will begin to do so. Suppose all technical people agree to be paid in Frika? Suppose all African states as they are today agree with the international community that all NGOs and Charities operating in Africa must have offices and bases in Central African Republic (CAR)? This may be the beginning of the CAR becoming the Federal Capital Territory of the Continental Union Government. Is this a plan that the CAR government is likely to accept? Such a plan may see the population of the area tripling in 10 years, but the whole economy completely transformed. I see in the CAR alone, at least a million new jobs and re-training opportunities for Africa's growing unemployed university graduates who are happy to relocate to the CAR if Africa is re-membered and the suggestions in this letter acted on. How many people are employed by the Chinese Government to administer 1.3 billion people? The UK National Health Service employs about a million people to provide health services for about 62 million people. Taking the existing manpower of individual African federal entities of today, we can begin to extrapolate the manpower needs of our superstate. Value creation is linked to wealth creation and the new AU stands to become possibly the greatest value creation in modern times. The employment opportunities will be massive! This AU enterprise with adequately trained manpower for a meticulous bureaucratic machinery and military precision will deliver the results if there is political will and an agreement with the international community. O Barack, this must be something completely new and unique to the needs of the continent and every pre-existing institution will need to adjust accordingly, for the innovation and change that the new AU would have become.

In the dreams above, I have hinted on the issue of reparations being paid to each African to begin the "accounting for everyone" process and the common currency. I am talking about reparations to Africa for European exploitations of the past and not reparations for slavery, which will for ever be impossible to pay for and will not make a difference to the "altered DNA" that resulted from slavery. Reparations for Africa is a controversial subject, but I sincerely believe that some official acknowledgement of the damage done to Africa through some payments designated as reparations will help the healing process, and remove some victimism-related excuses from our psyche especially if done with the pan-African innovations suggested above. How much exactly should be paid? How about $1,000 per person over 10 years? This is not a ridiculous figure as it amounts to $100 per person per year and a trillion dollars over the period, when $60 trillion has already been spent globally on aid over the last 60 years. Well, looking at it closely, it is the equivalent of the current flow of aid for only 20 years. In that case, should the reparation amount be $10,000 per person over the same period? I cannot say, but no one should imagine debt write offs and "forgiveness" as reparations! It reminds me of the carting away of artefacts from the ancient Benin Empire being seen in

70

some quarters as reparations for the killing of 7 white men in 1897. All debt so far to sham states are, without sounding ungrateful, sham debts as well! As far as I am aware, Itsekiri (my true nation) owes nobody or country any debt. If anything, we are owed billions of dollars by the oil companies and their collaborators who have between themselves shared our land and oil, taken away our fishing industry by polluting our waters, and collaborated with "governments" and the evil ones amongst us to kill Itsekiri people. Sham debts return to the lenders ultimately via corrupt leaders, Swiss banks, etc. This is why the common currency and its international controls will help curb corruption and capital flight. All these imagined, but put aside, the most important support will be for the international community to agree on a concerted plan to support the Frika. If well supported, the Frika could generate additional GDP and values in the minds of all players well above the current $1.5 trillion for the whole continent. For example if we agree that all major infrastructural projects, as far as is reasonably practicable, must have their raw materials sourced from the continent and paid for with the Frika, this will add value to the Frika. I certainly do believe that the common currency cannot only come into existence quicker than anticipated, but also holds the key to the acceleration of both political and economic developments. If the Earth's landmass was made of Africa only, would we not be self-sufficient? Prior to the "discovery" of Africa, were we not self-sufficient in our own primitive ways? We did not ask anyone for help. Outsiders came to disturb our "ecology" (to contrast the now more favourable word "economy") and expectations and began to exploit us in the process. When will this stop? Self-sufficiency boils down to people and their will. In the case of Africa, a schizophrenic illness brought on by the slave trade and colonisation has rendered the continent's mind (metaphoric economic development software) impotent and the soul unable to care for the body/flesh . . . observed roaming the earth with one hand, one leg and rags for clothing (the Negro in the Dutch colony seen by Voltaire's Candide). Indeed the human schizophrenics I saw as a child, in Nigeria looked just like this, with no government that truly cares.

The seeds of Special Administrative Arrangements (SAAs) in Africa growing to correct faulty foundations

If this letter is to be shredded or dismissed, this part must not be, O Barack. For all the ideas for a solution can be centred on the single concept of "Special Administrative Arrangements." Paul Collier, in his book *The Bottom Billion*, noted that export processing zones offer good use for aid money, and will promote economic growth whilst offering some protection against the traps that "bottom billion countries" tend to find themselves in. Dambisa Moyo in her book *Dead Aid*, prophetically saw a quasi-Utopia in Africa she named The Republic of Dongo – a hypothetical African state that will not rely on aid and grow economically. Even the baby AU, with some premonition, has proposed Special Economic Zones (SEZ), so I conclude that "the spirit s in the air". It does not really matter what we call these imagined and proposed places of intense economic activities, but one thing stands out if they will succeed – their administration.

There is no point giving incompetent people, born of nepotism, the task of administering our Utopia. This is why the term **Special Administrative Arrangement** and the acronym **SAA** is used in this letter. Without the birth of pockets of water-tight 21st century administrative processes in the form of SAAs, all over Africa, psychopathic corruption and incompetence will kill Dongo in 10 to 15 years (Dambisa should take note) and drink his blood. Without renewing or setting aside a lot of the minds in governments of Africa

72

today, another round of regression will be the natural outcome in a few years' time. *The leopard does not get rid of its spots*, says an African proverb. Knowing how rampant psychopathic corruption and incompetence are in Africa at the moment, and how difficult it is to unseat a seating but incompetent African "leader," only a negotiated lease of a piece of his country, by the AU will prevent him from taking his people down with him. His people, instead of risking death by crossing the Mediterranean ocean in a rickety boat to Europe will move to our SAA a few hundred miles from his home.

Not too long ago, I had a meeting with an English/UK business consultant who coincidentally had spent some of his youth in Nigeria. His parents had to leave their rubber plantation in 1967 following the outbreak of war in Nigeria that year. We discussed the idea of a Hong-Kong type of Special Administrative Region (SAR) in Nigeria which will ultimately result in the building of a brand new "21st century city" in Nigeria. One of his first and blunt questions to me was "what will potential investors say, when told *here is this great entrepreneurial project with Dr Temi Metseagharun, a psychiatrist behind it*"? Clearly, no one would take it seriously, I admitted. I also had candid discussions with other Nigerians including a young Nigerian entrepreneur and master's degree holder in finance. He was working as a nursing assistant in the UK, basically to raise funds for his investments back home. *"No, I don't think it is realistic,"* was the Nigerian's candid opinion regarding any grand entrepreneurial project related to a united African federal entity.

However, it is interesting to note that the older and more experienced European business consultant with vast experience in the Far East and Middle East did ask hard and sometimes discouraging questions, but actually felt the idea was perfectly realistic and proposed to invite his associates who have long experience in SARs, most notably Hong-Kong and Macau. He has since drawn out a 10 year timeline for the

73

city and it is not cash we are worried about, but how to get a powerful mentor with enough political muscle and how to creatively push through what we now call an SAA. Hopefully in Nigeria we will overcome the phenomenon of government officials asking *"how much is my cut?"* for any good and people-empowering idea to be implemented. I realised how important it is to share a vision with those with experience who want to see you succeed. People without any global vision of their own, cannot give guidance in this area and can only attempt to maintain the status quo or what they are familiar with. Upon further analysis, we realised that a "Special Administrative Region" to be leased from any African "country" or sovereign entity for 99 years as was the case of Hong-Kong, will today raise a lot of questions and suspicions, but not if the economic benefits are clearly visible to all concerned. At one point in my discussions with the consultant, it was the migration issues, as it happened in the middle days of Hong-Kong, that became an issue. Should we fence the area? How can we control people's movement into a part of their own country? Now we know that the migration issues within the AU will not be an issue if the EU radically revises its immigration laws and invests in AU new cities instead – this will help redirect migration away from Europe. After all, if it is greener pastures migrants are looking for, why not lease pieces of lands in their home continent and make them green? In reality, it is not the land that is green, but the mind-related political environment of freedom, meritocracy, kindness and human rights that make Europe "green" compared to Africa. It is my understanding of the "**African mind**" that I believe allows me to see creative solutions to the mind-related problems of Africa. All the ingredients for at least 3 brand new "21st century cities" are there in Nigeria, but little or no vision and incompetent "leaders" prevent the people from seeing the opportunity, not to talk of seizing it. It is the minds of human beings that make lands green. Give the land and all the money on earth to the wrong people or minds and nothing good will come out of it, but to the right people, the land surely will become greener. The reality of the possibility of a new Hong-Kong in Nigeria was strengthened by the observation that whereas the old Hong-Kong involved a lease from one sovereign country to another, a lease made to a profit-making company could see the company with the right European backing turn over cash like a country. Investors where are you? *"This will surely be setting a precedent if the 'arrangement' can be agreed,"* the consultant noted. With further discussions, we now agree that whilst capitalism will certainly be the driver of a good cash turnover, the lease ideally will be to another sovereign entity – the new AU, but the cities would still be profit-making and administered by a corporation.

The core idea of Special Administrative Arrangements is about using a combination of top-down and bottom-up approaches to build pockets of civil societies from scratch. The top-down approach should be about giving funds and assistance to a politically stronger AU and not to individual governments, whilst the bottom-up approach is via a few new continental cities (SAAs or SARs) dotted strategically across the continent.

O Barack, all you need do is put your name on these seeds . . . SARs as "Obama cities" in Africa – Special Administrative Areas with rock-solid socially-coherent foundations, free from Africa's past in terms of values and culture, but consistent with the advanced 21st century life and values, elsewhere in the Western world.

I have said it before and I will say it again: Talks of "neo-colonialism" are the preferred arguments of those who do not wish Africa well, and those who want to maintain the status quo that is to their advantage. If neo-colonialism was an issue, we would not have desperate Africans crossing the Mediterranean ocean and risking their lives to be under "colonial rule." Indeed any African, who talks seriously about neo-colonialism in my opinion, is retrogressive, if not hateful. The remnants of colonialism and neo-colonialism are in the form of despots and sham governments. A truly united Africa means the end of any form of neo-colonialism. Continental cities free of the administrative incompetence of despots and corrupt "leaders" can only be a refuge for the masses, the fatherless, the stateless and (thank goodness) those unemployed youths with skills, faith, passion, energy and courage that their "governments" care not about.

In a letter to the business consultant I mentioned in this letter, I gave the example of an SAR in Central African Republic (CAR) and not in Nigeria. CAR has a population of less than 5 million, but centrally located for administrative and logistic purposes. CAR is "pure Africa" with its animals, savannah vegetation, political problems and very high dependence on aid. It has land and rivers to support an SAA and the sort of economic growth that the right minds would produce even in the absence of abundant natural resources. I mentioned how such an SAA would be a creative solution to immigration and emigration problems as they affect Europe and Africa respectively. Europe's politicians will do well to radically revise their "asylum and immigration" principles.

My African refugee patients agree with me that if only the "billions" spent on immigration detention centres, immigration appeal lawyers and services were all based in an SAR in Africa, such an investment will be saving 100 birds with one nest – genuinely providing refuge without dehumanizing fellow humans in the name of immigration control. It is a shame to have a brave 25-year old woman risking her life by crossing the Mediterranean ocean, only to end up in an immigration detention centre. What a waste of human resources all because on the one side politicians hold on to out-dated principles and on the other side, the rulers simply don't care! We, Africans in Europe, are mostly economic migrants, and even if we are not, an SAR with standards of living no different from that of Europe will offer political asylum as well. Money spent on Immigration is similar to charity money being spent on Africa, but not in Africa. How nice will it be for all African charity and NGO consultants to compulsorily have their base in the SAA in Central African

Republic? That is probably 5 jobs per consultant created for the locals! How nice will it be for major universities all over the world to have campuses in SARs in Africa? The number and types of potential contributors, besides governments to proposed SAAs in Africa is limitless. SAAs can also bring about genuine "green revolutions" administered by Western experts, not incompetent and corrupt governments. With SAAs dotted all over Africa and the help of "Zimbabwean farmers," the AU will be self-sufficient in food.

I was having a chat with a colleague of mine about the humanitarian needs of Africa. He wasted no time in telling me that he was concerned and that for a few years now, he has been sponsoring a goat. He carefully explained how this small contribution really helps the villagers where the goat is. This was 4 years ago, and I still don't know what to make of this humanitarian gesture. All I can say is that sponsoring a goat seems like a good idea, but not one that the "African mind" that I know of can relate to. What about microfinance credit? I suppose that given the messianic work of Muhammad Yunus and Grameen bank, we expect a replication of the Bangladeshi experience in Africa. Again, I can state confidently that the "African Mind" that I know of will see bank microfinance credit as institutional money.

In Nigeria, institutional money is generally seen as nobody's money, and therefore there will be little or no accountability from within on the part of managers and receivers. The African mind that I know of has an ego made of lead! He may be poor, but he would want to go on shopping in Europe or Dubai, stay in 5-star hotels and drive the biggest SUVs, BMWs and Mercedes for his neighbours to see. His community may have little or no infrastructure, but so long as he has his "palace," he is happy. Out of the mentality of the people arises that of their leaders. The lifestyles of some African rulers, such as the Swazi King, and Nigerian "legislators," tell the story. Nigerian legislators are the highest paid in the world – over $ 1 million per annum; plus bribes. I saw with my own eyes a long list of Nigerian officials who have bought properties and time share in Dubai whilst Nigeria suffers from infrastructural decay. **Why don't we create a Dubai and a little piece of Europe in Nigeria?** I asked myself. This way at least, whilst feeding our frivolities, we could prevent capital flight and provide employment opportunities for the people, thereby increasing their standard of living. Knowing full well how my brethren love luxury, I know that their egos will pay for it even in Nigeria. Making a small piece of Nigeria no different from Western Europe means giving 150 million people access to the perceived luxury in Europe without a visa. How come no one sees this business opportunity? Now we know it is feasible and the funds are there in the pockets of Nigerians! The question however is who will do it? With the principle of converting only small pieces of land to be no different from Western Europe, we can expect the same standards of administration, infrastructure, medical care, education and luxury – the strongest psychological pull for African rulers and elites. For this, an SAR or SAA and a minimum lease period of 50 years are required. Otherwise, standards of administration and the very "African mind" problems will get us back to the norm. The good thing here and the expectation is that before the lease is over, the Union Government of the AU would have become strong enough and despots will have no role to play anymore in the continent. Other administrative boundaries may have come into effect with the tribal house and senate making decisions based on the authenticity of representation. Also, Africa expects the return of hundreds of thousands of high net worth Africans from all over the world to the continent; and with continental cities with standards no different from those of Western Europe, potential returnees should join this enterprise and have a ready-made bed for retirement back in Africa. I believe I already know several people who are looking to return, but have nowhere "proper" to return to. They need a dream home in their homeland. Hindsight and foresight are the ingredients in my meditations

O Barack. SARs are not new (hindsight) and SAAs will be marvellous (foresight).

Other aspects of the true African Union

It is important to acknowledge that that the baby AU as it is today is fairly sophisticated, but needs more grassroots involvement and less "heads of state" involvement! This will require social engineering using 21st century technology as already proposed. Other aspect can be summarised as follows: **European immigration systems and laws:** *"A human tsunami,"* says Silvio Berlusconi, the Italian prime minister in distress as Italy's Island of Lampedusa becomes the temporary home of impoverished illegal immigrants from Africa. *"It's time for good immigration and not mass migration,"* says David Cameron, the UK's prime minister at about the same time as Silvio Berlusconi, but much far away from Lampedusa and protected from the human tsunami and the rest of Europe by the English Channel. Good talk. But are these leaders addressing the deeper and fundamental reasons for migration? How about stemming emigration? How about re-evaluating the principles of political asylum? How about re-considering immediate movement to a safe and humane location and accommodation away from the EU - avoiding the word "deportation" - whenever anyone presents themselves in any part of Europe without valid documents? Immigration remains a thorny issue for Europe, and requires a radical overhaul, but it seems there is a lack of political will to take the issue head on; perhaps due to the soft political left misunderstanding the needs of migrants. However, the new, stronger and capitalised AU will offer the EU a wonderful opportunity to overhaul her immigration principles, philosophy and rules to meet the migration realities of the modern world in the 21st century. Europe may be faced with the risks of serious, potentially disastrous and irreparable integration problems and problems with religion and race relations if immigration is not appropriately controlled and even capped as some have advised. For the sake of economic refugees like me, I cannot support a cap, but I will gladly do so if the cap comes with shifting the EU "joint immigration headquarters" to an SAA in North Africa with a "Mediterranean beach resort"! This is serious talk. Twice, my wife and I had to pay for her younger brother (the only one of 8 siblings who, due to funny immigration rules, is not a British citizen) who lives in Yemen, to go over to North Africa to enable family members to see him. The first time was to Algeria and the next time was to Sharm-El-Sheik in Egypt, and the beach experience was good. It is worth noting that despite winning in an Immigration Appeals Tribunal, my wife's brother was not given a visa. He almost camped out at the British Embassy asking for his visa, but he was told *"Yes, we will give you the visa, but we'll call you when we get the papers from the UK."* Two years on, he has not been contacted and will not be contacted like several other people that we came to find out about. So what is the point of having an Immigration Appeals Tribunal whose decisions will simply be ignored? Why is tax payer's money being wasted on a kangaroo "appeals tribunal"? Well, as an indirect form of collective justice, it is understandable as to why in 2009, no young Yemeni would be given a visa to the UK, if they had never travelled to the EU before. Indeed, the rule in 2007 was close to this description, given Al Qaida's presence in Yemen. As someone who is now familiar with Middle Eastern culture I can say confidently that it will be a grave mistake for the EU not to radically review its immigration principles. My advice to Europe: Do not destroy yourselves in the process of holding on to out-dated political asylum and immigration principles. Do not cut the immigration-related budgets of Europe, but divert the cash, the work, the buildings and other infrastructure and personnel all to our SAA. The SAA will provide the very jobs that unemployed youths are seeking in Europe. Surely, Europe does not want to continue with another form of *"I'll pay myself to help you"* type of shambolic exercise in the name of immigration control and "appeals tribunal". With a bit of innovation and creativity, other people can enjoy the pleasure of multiculturalism like I am certainly doing as a Christian married to a Muslim; Nigerian married to an Arab and we are a British family by nationality.

I have lost count of the number of times I have had to help people with immigration issues, and with my experience comes a frustration with unhelpful rules, waste of human resources, and adherence to out-dated rules that are simply exploited by those who ideally should not have been allowed into the country in the first place. I have helped to pay for people to actually voluntarily leave the UK without the pressure of immigration authorities. They realised that Europe was not for them, and that the "soft immigrants" are ruthlessly dealt with, whist the hard ones manipulate the rules, get into fake marriages, identity fraud, etc., to beat the system. *Why should they deport a man in a love marriage with children, and in the same week grant political asylum to plane hijackers?* My cousin asked me. I challenge EU policy makers to prove that they are not only good at dealing with the softies. Europe will do the AU a lot of good if a pan-European immigration law stipulates that all asylum seekers should be housed in an AU-EU SAR in Africa. If asylum is the real issue, then what could possibly be wrong with a part of Africa that is no different from Western Europe, standards-wise? Just like I immigrated to Europe, so did some of my fellow doctors from Nigeria to the only SAA in Africa until 1994 – South Africa.

Unification and centralisation of African Aid provisions.

This is the "market" of NGOs, charitable organisations and the "aid industry": They must, just like the global bankers and mobile telecommunications experts referred to earlier, take advantage of the benefits of a truly unified Africa. As mentioned already, a way of doing this is to agree by a United Nations charter and other laws and in principle, that all NGOs and charities operating in any part of Africa must have a base in Central African Republic (our proposed new federal capital territory). There will be the benefit of pulled resources, central coordination and of course prioritisation and reduction of duplications and conflicting ideas on how good should be done. Paul Collier, in his book *The Bottom Billion* gave an example of 3 charities attempting to build a school and ended up with the ridiculous suggestion of building separate floors without working together! It seems they have caught up with the shambolic governments of Africa! Another way that aid provision can help the unification of Africa is for all technocrats to agree to be paid in Frika. This way, Africa will probably attract only those who really care about the continent and not those who want to use charities to enrich their pockets and in reality do little for the continent. Africa needs incarnates of the likes of Mary Slessor. Come and live with us and adopt our children without taking them to a foreign land and away from their siblings and cause a furore in the media.

Merging of African debt and lending processes.

The fact that the West and now China give cash to African "governments" is one of my most worrying observations in African affairs. I hate to come across as a believer in popular conspiracy theories, but why would anybody give cash to an unrepresentative government, if the giver does not have a sinister agenda against the people? Emerging Powers: Africa's New Exploiters? That is the question Jean-Michel Severino and Oliver Ray asked as a chapter in their book, *Africa's Moment.* My answer is YES THEY ARE! I thought capitalism is fundamentally about allowing the people and not their government to control capital and that communism is the opposite. So, why are supposedly capitalist governments turning to communism when it comes to Africa? Will Africa not be better off having private firms and individuals lent cash (capital) instead of their governments? Will the tax system, transparency and accountability of these "countries" not be better off with capital going directly to entrepreneurs and specific projects? Indeed, if General Sani Abacha of Nigeria or another African dictator, who stole or misappropriated oil or Aid money had been personally (and not Nigeria as a nation), loaned $10 Billion for a specific project, I am sure the West would not have problems getting back the cash and Abacha's assets from Switzerland (a country that persistently refuses to return stolen cash from Africa). The freezing of private terrorist-linked funds is the proof of lack of political will by Western leaders to lend responsibly and retrieve Africa's stolen wealth. Perhaps it is a good thing that the political will had been delayed until an auspicious time as now, where with the new AU, the recovered funds will not simply be misappropriated or stolen again. When lending processes don't hold individuals accountable, they simply allow the contractor to abandon the project and enjoy his loot. The sad thing is that the ordinary people collectively are then held responsible for the actions of a single individual who never truly represented them in the first place. Again, even in the corporate world, banks hardly lend money to small companies unless the directors offer personal guarantees which mean that should the companies fail, the directors' assets will be liquidated. This should be an incentive for the company directors to ensure that the company succeeds, and a disincentive to misappropriate or embezzle corporate funds.

It is little wonder it has been estimated that as much of 40% of military spending in some sham states comes from aid money, which tragically implies loans, aid and donations funding useless unprofessional armies to kill the people and abuse their rights. My worry here is a serious one, because when the corrupt government misappropriate, embezzles or simply waste the money, the people are then held responsible indirectly and suffer the consequences whilst the "leader" and his family smile all the way to a Swiss bank account. And the givers? What happens to them? Well they usually get about 30% (or more) return on their investments and enjoy the benefits of "I'll pay myself to help you" type of medicine to the dying man. In my opinion, most of the cash spent on Africa by Europe goes back to Europe or Europeans eventually, and China may now be attempting to milk that European cash indirectly through trade, by flooding African markets with cheap goods where the European version of the same goods cannot compete in our "manufacturing-free" consumer markets.

This is an area where I am in no position to say much. All I can say is that all African debt till date is largely part of the sham governing of the continent. The new Africa must be born debt-free! I cannot imagine a situation where I will become responsible for my father's debt. I, like all humans was born naked, owning or owing nothing, but dependent on the love and goodwill of others. So should be the case of the new Africa. But my parents did feed me, educated me and put me on a course of self-sufficiency and independence without my inheriting any cash. This should be how the future of our new Africa must be until it reaches the hypothetical age of adulthood, when it can take on its own debt only after proving itself reasonably internally self-sufficient. Again, the lenders, IMF and World Bank, are the experts here (in their market) to decide how the common currency can be used as a means to tidy up the debt and lending processes of incompetent states. I anticipate that since the value of all cash is a function of the human mind, then all hands should be on deck to ensure that the currency maintains its value through creative means such as trading oil, diamonds and other minerals in Frika and having all capital projects in Africa for the next 2 decades to be agreed in principle and by law to be paid in Frika. Here the Chinese could really help out and have a bit of currency reserve in Africa!

In merging the debt and lending process of the entire continent, no African government should henceforth be loaned any cash. Whatever they need the cash for is probably best done as a private enterprise where value for money will be judged, and all workers will pay taxes from which the government will fund itself and the people will demand accountability for the money taken from them that their eyes can see and their pockets can feel. Yes, from the provision of health facilities and schools to the construction of roads, I cannot see why private firms cannot be loaned the cash. The little known, but very rich German construction company, Julius Berger, that operates in Nigeria is known to facilitate the treatment of Nigerian presidents in Nigeria and in Germany. Why? Well, that is an indirect theft of Nigeria's oil money through construction projects with over-inflated cost! Part of the benefit of having Julius Berger in Nigeria, is better health care in an oil rich country that benefits the Government, but not the people. In an aid-dependent "country," there will be absolutely no justification to give the cash for such projects to the government. All loan-supported capital projects should be through the AU. With the AU's new power, capitalisation and sophistication, such projects will be supervised and made absolutely transparent by the AU government to prevent

85

kickbacks and other forms of corruption, incompetence and inefficiency that kill capital projects in Africa. Now what problem could a local (colonial state) government have with this arrangement? The project is for the people, the government will tax the companies and the workers and the people will be required to pay other justifiable levies to their government. What could possibly be to the disadvantage of the government except for snatching away the cookies from thieves?

Unified anti-corruption organisation (Police force)

It is all about corruption! . . . . psychopathic corruption.

With Africa's unique form of corruption that sometimes involve the occult, only a powerful, legitimate pan-African anti-corruption organisation, free from the influence of any president, incompetence, corruption (O yes, corruption in a supposedly anti-corruption body), ethnic bias and lack of sustainability, can stem this most powerful demon in Africa.

Nowhere else on Earth I believe, are there better examples of shambolic anti-crime organisations like Nigeria's EFCC, Economic and Financial Crimes Commission. Its sister organisation, ICPC, Independent Corrupt Practices and Other Related Offences Commission, has had only a handful of convictions since its inception over 10 years ago, despite the country being riddled with official corruption! Like I mentioned earlier, the more it looks like the real thing, the more a sham is a sham. To go into the activities of Nigeria's EFCC is to write another book, but "wikileaked" cables show how much Nigerian government officials themselves agree that the organisation is a sham. It would not be too troublesome if the shambolic process did not have teeth; but it does and the teeth is used only to bite enemies of the president and some "collateral damage" as part of making the sham look like the real thing. For every person persecuted by Nigeria's

86

EFCC, there are a thousand government thieves and fraudsters in need of prosecution. What can one expect when the government itself is a fraud? Interestingly, there is a well-written document on a pan-African fight against corruption – AFRICAN UNION CONVENTION ON PREVENTING AND COMBATING CORRUPTION (2003) - sitting on the shelves and gathering dust for obvious reasons. Now, let us assume that the U.S, EU and China agree to offer $10 billion for the setting up and running of the AU's pan-continental unified anti-corruption organisation in the form of a police force, with the caveat that all governments must sign up to a process of transparency and prosecution of all government and company or corporate corruption by the African court of Justice. Well, the people will sign up in a referendum, but not the governments and certainly not Nigeria's EFCC. The sum of $10 billion looks quite huge and I suppose at this point readers of this letter may have become a bit cynical of my tendency to mention huge sums of cash, as if I have them myself or could conjure them from the heavens. I anticipate that some readers could sarcastically say that perhaps, I really do believe in conspiracy theories of how bankers create money from thin air in the process of fractional reserve lending, etc. Or perhaps, I really do believe in my understanding of the human mind to the point where I "know" that gold is in the land, but money is in the mind only! $10 billion is the amount estimated to leave Africa yearly through corruption, so I do not believe my mention of such an amount is unreasonable.

Away from this digression, realistically, what will $10 billion do for a pan-African police force that begins life as an anti-corruption organisation for the continent? In my opinion, it will revolutionise the police forces in Africa and governance in the whole of the world if the rest of the world cooperates. Yes, there is no error in the preceding statement as governance in the rest of the world permits "soft corruption" in the form of Swiss-type banks and Halliburton-like multi-national companies. Sadly, "soft corruption" in the West fosters very

87

hard and callous corruption backed by impunity in Africa. Nigeria's Halliburton corruption scandal is a perfect example of how "soft corruption" in the West diminishes good governance even in the West. For those who are not familiar with the Halliburton case, it is worth noting that Halliburton systematically bribed Nigerian government officials with at least $300 million to enable the company procure a lucrative contract to build a multi-billion dollar liquefied natural gas plant. The company has since been prosecuted in the U.S and fined $300 million, but absolutely nothing besides a facade prosecution is going on in Nigeria . . . and then . . . the former vice president of the United States of America, Dick Cheney was threatened with prosecution by Nigeria's sham anti-corruption organisation. A lot of us thought it was a joke, but guess what? Dick Cheney paid up! What is the interpretation? Halliburton alone has just provided over half a billion - in fines and recoverable assets - of our $10 billion to get the pan-African anticorruption agency cracking . . . if only there is political will O dear Barack.

We will not go into the truth that it is the people of Africa and the Niger Delta that global soft corruption and Halliburton have robbed and the fact that we pay with sorrow, tears and blood for Western soft corruption. Yes, I mentioned the all-important word "political will" O Barack. In reality, the pan-African anti-corruption police force/organisation does not really need $10 billion from the U.S, EU and china. All it needs is urgent global/international, UN-led legislation stipulating that the pan-African anti-corruption organisation should take all recovered funds for itself for the next decade. I am sure it will raise half a trillion dollars in recovered funds and fines in a short time, and the next question will be what to do with such a huge amount of funds. Will that not threaten its integrity? No, I say, if the organisation is not a sham. Shams are usually built from faulty foundations and this is why, with the benefits of our current hind- and foresights, we will effectively create a system that largely bypasses human faults

88

and weaknesses by calling on the spirit of Daniel chapter 2 verse 45: . . . the vision of the rock cut out of a mountain, but not by human hands—a rock that broke the iron, the bronze, the clay, the silver and the gold to pieces. If it is principle-centred ("not cut by human hands"), completely transparent as in being "online and real-time" wherever possible without compromising operational issues and have no human "head," then it will not be a sham. But how can an organisation not have a head? Of course there will be a mind, but not a head. This is not new as countless numbers of institutions do not have human heads, they just have a mind (personality and culture), built by the "founding fathers" and the human heads, which from time to time seem to be at the head, are like executive cells of the brain that can by no means represent the human mind, which is always a whole in its mode of functioning. In practice, this may involve the democratization of a large organisation, with each chief executive doing no more than 6 months at a time and each board member not more than 2 years and being prepared to go back to the frontline of policing and prosecution. It is the rotation and dynamism at the top that will mean that one human head cannot foster its agenda on the rest and that ultimately, only the principles will survive and potentially into eternity (Daniel 2:44 - It will crush all those kingdoms and bring them to an end, but it will itself endure forever), unless a critical change in the environment necessitates an "amendment of the constitution."

The initial mode of funding is likely to be very aggressive and adversarial since it is partly driven by organisational self-interest (funding linked to successful prosecutions), but it will be for a limited time. Unlike Nigeria's sham EFCC, the organisational thinking will be...

"why should I accept a bribe from you corrupt miscreant when I can take all your ill-gotten money for myself? Besides, I will look towards keeping you in jail and out of circulation

for a long time so that you do not attempt to corrupt my members. "

Like any deep thinking individual, I will be careful not to create a self-serving organisation, but if the extra funds raised are directed towards funding and training the entire police forces in Africa, then revolution of the police forces in Africa will indeed come to pass as stated above. It would be interesting to see how the dynamics of the continental and national police forces pan out; for creativity demands that a "council of national police forces" should be given the power to sack the board of the continental force at any time, barring all or some previous board members from contesting the next round of elections. I suppose this will ensure that should no "excess cash" trickle downwards, the board better be prepared to have a reason acceptable to the Pan-African Court of Justice. With so many stake holders and internal regulatory processes, I do not envisage that one governor or even a president can bribe his/her way out of prosecution. Besides, if the organisation is proactive, for example, requesting from all levels of government and public organisations, measures of transparency and due process in all spending, I am sure a lot of corruption will be prevented. There will also be the "side effect" of good accounting all over Africa. Is this just a dream? No, not if there is political will, O Barack. Again, if the organisation has no restrictions on nationalities for the first 5 years and provides good pay and housing in Central African Republic, at least in the initial phase that will involve global recovery of loot, then it should attract the talents and conscience of the world.

Unified and single electoral body

This has already been discussed, but it is worth noting that such a body, like a common anti-corruption police force will reduce drastically the occurrence of electoral fraud that produces fraudulent governments and shambolic incompetent criminals who pose as representatives of the people. With appropriate data coming from our continental census, combined with appropriate technology, voting on paper (physical voting) should turn out to be ceremonial and a kind of formality, given that the technology would allow pin-controlled remote electronic voting as well.

Unified Army and single permanent peace-keeping force

I dare say that even Egypt does not require its own army under the control of its president. Why not? The relevant question is army for what? Is it to fight Israel? This act will amount to a suicidal gesture. Is it to fight Libya or to fight for other Arab countries? Or as it happens all over Africa, to be used to oppress and kill the very people they purport to defend?! Whatever Egypt needs an army for, the Northern divisions of the unified African force will be in a better position to carry out professionally and dispassionately. As a matter of fact, an Egypt without its own army makes the Israeli-Palestinian conflict less likely to ever result in a major war, and liberates the people of Egypt from having any more despotic pharaohs in modern times. Indeed, the AU (in the form of its predecessor – the OAU) took sides with Egypt and most of its member countries broke off diplomatic relationships with Israel in the 1970s. The stronger and truly unified AU's role in the peace process therefore cannot be underestimated. It may turn out to become one of the surest routes to a no appetite for war against Israel. The cradle of human evolution and civilisation - Africa – having "the lands of scripture" and faith as its friendly neighbours, could be the beginning of a new era for humanity. Now if Egypt with Africa's largest Army does not require one, what about Nigeria or Guinea? Agreed, the Nigerian army has not recently been accused of raping its own citizens like the Guineans did, and the Congolese are still doing till date, but they did not only massacre civilians in the Biafra war, they did rape the people. Their intrusion into

91

Nigeria's politics only accelerated the decline of a promising experiment. Their activities in the Niger Delta is interesting; sometimes they kill the locals, but to be fair to them they are trying to be professional and are now more concerned about thieving in collaboration with the "governments" and local militia. What a sham!

Also the immediate constitution of a well-paid continental army that first admits rebels and soldiers alike from conflict zones is likely to remove combatants from the scenes, bringing an almost immediate relief to the people in the process. So many unemployed youths will benefit from the discipline of military service without war. Also, what a wonderful opportunity it will be to retrain Africa's youths, especially the ones with weapons masquerading as armies, rebels or freedom fighters. Indeed, a whole army of very helpful and economically positive farmers and construction workers could come out of a highly disciplined and professional 21st century army for Africa. O Barack no country needs a useless and completely unprofessional army in the 21st century!

Unified and single Tourism board

North Africa, South Africa and parts of East Africa are doing fairly well, but will do better by pulling resources together. West Africa is not doing well and one look at Nigeria's tourism board and their "master plan" shows how shambolic the board is. Yes, they called in a consultant, but what did they do with the advice of the consultant? What are they doing about sales and marketing? What are they doing about necessary infrastructure? What are they doing about reputation of the country and insecurity? How many Nigerians return yearly with friends and family from all over the world? Where do they stay and where do they visit? I guess at this point I may have used the word "sham" a hundred times, so I will say nothing about Nigeria's tourism industry. Only a unified African Tourism Board can direct curiosity to the most populous country with black-skinned people on earth; the savannahs and game reserve in Northern Nigeria and down south, the forests of the Niger delta and the historical drummers of the coast of West Africa. Perhaps only the presence of an SAA (Special Administrative Arrangement) can make tourism a viable industry in Nigeria. I speak of Nigeria's wasting of potential because that is the place I am most familiar with. A unified tourism board will link the Safaris of Kenya to the Savannah belt of West Africa opening new markets in the process. The same board will link the beach holidays of North Africa to the currently non-existent beach holidays in the coast of West Africa. Who will market and sell the road from Cape Town to Cairo? I certainly consider it a lifetime dream to move across the continent from south to north by road or by rail over a 2 week period in one year and then from west to east in another year. "Continental roads" – 6-lane "tourists roads and rail lines" from Cape Town to Cairo and from Banjul (The Gambia) to Cape Guadarfui (Somalia) punctuated by "stop zones" every 100 – 200 miles can be imagined easily as part of infrastructural development that will stimulate the local economy by providing jobs and income with tourist paying in Frika. "Stop zones" can be imagined as service stations, but much bigger as the nucleus of new small and highly secure towns with decent hotels for people from all over the world. Of course, it is easy to dream and sometimes build with the expectation that people will come, only to be faced with harsh realities once we start. Well, in this case I am very optimistic, because unless Africa retrogresses, with increase in leisure as the dream future of pleasure-seeking and prosperous mankind, tourism can only increase world-wide and will therefore be the biggest potential industry for Africa. We will be wise to not just dream, but take actual step to actualise the dream. You can do a "round the earth trip" and skip Africa, but you would have known and experienced nothing about the central landmass of planet earth!

Unified and single mineral resources board

Let us not beat about the bush here. We know that the return on investments in Africa is quite high simply because the people and their sham governments are exploited by mineral exploiting companies and their local collaborators. A disingenuous claim is that the higher returns are the rewards for high risk, but it does not change the fact that a mature adult taking advantage of a vulnerable pubertal teenager gives him or her satisfaction only when morality is thrown out of the window. The best example is provided by what is going on in the Niger Delta –Economic rape.

"Well, well," (I'm not going to listen to you) says the oil company. "You do benefit from the oil, don't you?" (You do derive pleasure from being raped, don't you?)

"No," I say. "but you and your co-rapists do"

The co-rapists are the middlemen in the mineral exploitation industry. The same middlemen are the individuals who occupy offices in shambolic governments. They are crooked officials who ultimately are products of wickedness, short-sightedness, cronyism, nepotism and other forms of corruption – interested only in their pockets. Crumbs fall for the people and help in building the existing sham mineral resources industry regulation. Most people are not aware, but at the same time the BP oil spill in the Gulf of Mexico was going on Exxon-Mobil had a similar spill in the Niger Delta. If the news is correct, absolutely nothing was done about it!

Nigeria's agony dwarfs the gulf oil spill – The Guardian

Nigeria: "World oil pollution capital" – BBC News

Niger delta oil spills dwarfs BP, Exxon Valdez catastrophes – neswdesk.org

This is rape O Barack . . . for you did not allow BP to take advantage of Americans, but there was nobody to stop Mobil from taking advantage of us! This is economic and

94

environmental rape! A quick look at the official website of the Nigerian Government (http://www.nigeria.gov.ng/) modelled on http://www.whitehouse.gov/issues may shed more light on Nigeria's handling of oil spills.

"To the people here in the Niger Delta, we are going to be standing by your side. And to Nigerians all across the country, come on down and visit."

Who made this statement on behalf of Nigerians?

Well, no one did and the statement above is yours O Barack, modified in the land of wishful thinking by imaging the Gulf of Mexico to be the Niger Delta. If you click on "Issues" in the official Nigerian Government website nothing comes up. Now you see an example of African Government ineptitude. O Barack, without a unified single mineral resources board for the whole of Africa, I cannot see how this rape will not continue. I will not talk about "blood diamonds" and the exploitation of the people and cassiterite of the Congo for over 100 years. All my common sense tells me is that divide and rule is still at work in Africa. The more divided we are, the easier it is for predators to make preys out of us . . . but as they say, unity is strength and more so if a great number of entities unite. Now I have to say that this board must be about fairness and not retribution; for although the pain of the exploitation so far may call for retribution, we shall rise above vengeance, open up a genuine truth and reconciliation committee and begin a new start with justice and fairness as the guiding principles.

Unified African law and The African Court of Justice

Nowhere else in the world is such a court so desperately needed. The European Court of Justice is now well-established and we all can see the benefits. All Africa needs is to slightly modify the European version along culturally sensitive lines, without removing the elements that amount to universal positive human values and rights – the very stone with which we intend to build our mountain. Such a functioning court and our new Continental police would begin an immediate governing of existing judiciaries all over Africa, guide new legislation (which must now be in line with the highest laws of the land) and ensure the independence and application of the principles of justice.

Unified parallel continental African Education programmes

Continental secondary schools and Continental Universities can spring up all over the continent if we agree that maintaining the highest standards of education is our desire. We can begin as soon as possible if we agree to convert all existing African Universities established before 1980 to "Continental Universities" responsible to the Union and not to individual states. I know how desperate some universities in Nigeria are to be relieved of the influence of their so-called chancellors who in the past have been uneducated and sometimes illiterate military generals who have no understanding of what universities are about, having not passed through such an institution. Nigerians will immediately understand what is being suggested here, as for decades Cameroonians crossed their western border to stream into Nigerian Universities. What an embarrassment I felt when my Cameroonian university mates were asked to go back home along with the rest of us after our university was shut down by the half-literate despotic general Sani Abacha for 9 months! In our continental universities and hopefully with our new AU, nothing like that will ever happen again. We will no longer have the madness of the gun ruling the places of learning, for the only weapon allowed in the battlefield of academia is the brain. Let those who have it not, never venture there in. I have to say at this point that I actually believe more in primary

96

education than university education because of its foundational aspects. A well-educated primary school graduate can continue with self-education outside the walls of a school and succeed in life. I strongly believe this, having seen it in close family members. My hope is that the advent of the ASSC (African Social Security Card) will help to creatively modernise and incentivise African primary education. In the wonderful world of my imagination, I imagine myself as a primary school teacher. O, that period of a child's life when seeds can be sowed and roots develop spontaneously. At one point during my primary school education, we had class rooms and teachers, but no furniture. As a 7 year old, I had to carry a chair and a desk to school every day for a period of time, but today I enjoy the returns of an investment in primary education. Today, sham states fail to bother to provide universal primary education. What a privilege it will be in our new Africa if we could guide the minds of the newest generation of the people who inhabit Africa! At this point philosophers will see another human being once again dreaming up a utopia, but the issue of education cannot be separated from direct and indirect concepts of Utopia. Well, let me have my ASSC, and leave the rest to God.

Unified healthcare and "Continental Hospitals"

At this point, a pattern should have been observed where the pooling together of resources and the reliefs from the shackles of sham governments can only improve services and standards. Continental hospitals can be imagined along the lines of continental universities described already with a selection of existing teaching hospitals being made continental centres of excellence, free from the shackles of maladministration of sham governments. African doctors and healthcare professionals and administrators are right there with the best of the world, but often not in Africa. Why? A lot of them had their initial training in Africa, but had to leave and were in no hurry to return. Why, when people in Africa are in desperate need of their services? It is not just about money, as crooked doctors are usually richer in Nigeria than their counterparts in the U.S. Besides, it is unlikely that people become very rich or good doctors if money was the main reason they chose medical practice as a profession. Healthcare in Africa is in a mess simply because sham governments do not really care. Why should any leader not develop his country's healthcare system to a point where he can rely on the services for his own health care? One good reason that a lot of people may not realise is key to this phenomenon, is that sham governments never genuinely invest in people. In the midst of corruption and nepotism, who will the government give a scholarship to train in the best Universities in the world, to acquire the necessary skills and come back home and serve? Well, it would suit the despot to send his relatives, but like him, the relative may be more interested in politics than medicine, and may not have the brain. So, the despot sends no one and when he is ill he goes abroad for treatment. Just as it is with manufacturing, whenever we can afford it, we would rather go abroad for manufactured goods instead of making a local product and developing it to become just as good as and even more accessible than the one abroad. There are numerous health-related NGOs and charities in Africa all in need of coordination and pooling of their resources in one base in the Central African Republic. With all those well-paid and experienced professionals working disparately all now coming together, the African Unified healthcare system could begin from there . . . and we could even have the equivalent of the UK's National Health Service. If we follow the sequence of execution of the True AU Project beginning with the continental census, then there will be no need for a special NHS number or card when the ASSC is already there. Health research will be improved with the improvement of the reliability of data. The benefits of a unified healthcare system for Africa are too numerous for me to go into . . . and as with other areas, I'll leave the debate and further meditation to those who know their market.

Unified and single continental economic development programme

African single market, subsidised agriculture and manufacturing as the continental route to economic growth:

Basically, Africa as it is today is a dumping ground for goods and "services"! In their book "Enough: Why the World's Poorest Starve in an Age of Plenty" Roger Thurow and Scott Kilman, discussed how the aid agencies bypassed Ethiopian-grown food right there in Ethiopia with warehouses full of grain at a time of need, allegedly to help the starving people of Ethiopia. The authors did in fact, use the word "schizophrenia" as a metaphor to describe what is going on in Africa without realising that it was no more metaphoric than the actual disease which is diagnosed purely based on symptoms. "Well, it serves me well to pay myself to help you." How about that? This is a disorder. Of course, Thurow and Kilman noted that the decision of where the food aid agencies must buy food from is made in line with U.S domestic needs and policies. Even Paul Collier noted that this is an area that is very shameful for Western countries that purport to want to help Africa, but subsidise their farming to make it impossible for African farmers to compete even in their own countries, talk less of Western countries. So basically, Africa provides employment for millions of other people all over the world as rich governments pay subsidies to their farmers and the IMF and World Bank prevents African "nations" from paying subsidies to their farmers. I suppose the issue here is one of initial self-sufficiency and capacity building up to a point, and then whatever else comes from abroad must be one of genuinely higher value. In our new AU, no food must be purchased from outside the AU as food aid except we are about to exhaust our stock. How much food do we require yearly in Africa? Why don't we set out to have enough stock to last several years from local farming? There is no doubt that Africa can feed itself: Thurow and Kilman have exhaustively written on the unfairness of trade against Africa and the ridiculous policies being forced down the throats of African governments; and there will be no need for me to go into it. It is worth noting that famine is not new to Africa or the Middle East. What happened in times of famine in pre-historic times was that people simply migrated like the children of Jacob did and went to Egypt. With the next famine, people would simple move (with their ASSCs) to the next geographical zone where there is no famine or they would visit the local food store a few miles away that accepts the ASSC. For now, all I can say is that with a single African food/commodities market, single currency and a single commodities/trade board, there should be guaranteed safe price for all farmers in our new Africa (strengthened AU); and with the advent of ASSC and freedom of movement across the existing "countries" of Africa, feeding camps will be a thing of the past. Surely, a single market consisting of a billion people holds a lot of potential. O Africa, you must unite! O Barack, you cannot afford not to be part of this African unity, and by making African unity a fundamental U.S foreign policy for Africa, the U.S will naturally become the closest and most trusted partner of (potentially) the next most important global player!

What about manufacturing and industrialisation?

The unified continent offers excellent opportunities for "forcing" in manufacturers. The problem with manufacturing not really taking off in Africa can be blamed on the "divide and rule" of foreign manufacturers. All the small African "countries" (representing Africa dismembered) can in no way compete against American, Japanese, European, and now Chinese and Indian manufacturing. Africa today is in a much worse situation than Asia in the 1930s and 40s, because the

100

cheap labour market in Asia is still there, and the "wage gradient" that should attract manufacturers to Africa is overshadowed by the political instability, poor infrastructure and economic sabotage of sham governments. However, with SAAs (Special Administrative Arrangements or Special Economic Zones under the AU) dotted all over Africa as part of the new AU, this obstacle would be bypassed and a new beginning would be the best opportunities for companies to expand their manufacturing. Now, how do we ensure that the common man of Africa benefits from the expected acceleration of manufacturing in the continent? In my mind, I have no doubt that African manufacturers and the emerging African middleclass market must be artificially protected. I'm sorry, but there must be no "free trade" with unequal partners in Africa! You must wait until we build our manufacturing and agricultural capacity. Here is the deal: All the companies who intend to sell their goods and services in Africa must join the process of our true African Union early enough for "limited monopoly rights" which are very much like patents. If you are willing to come in and invest now, then for the next 15 -20 years, we'll have you alone or you and only a few others. Remember, in another 50 years, Africa may have 2 billion (or even more) people before the culture of having less children catches up with us. At this rate, Africa will be the largest single market if we build up the middle class and manufacturing.

The need for special protection of the African Market

In his book *The Bottom Billion* Professor Collier discussed how the Structural Adjustment Programme (SAP) in Nigeria "worked" and how Nigerians perceive the opposite. I take this as an insult to Nigerians by a professor who is attempting to cover up his failure and the failure of the World Bank in their efforts to help growth and development. We are grateful for the help, but with all due respect to the professor, he did notice the shambolism of African "states" noting that *"Even the appearance of modern government in these states is sometimes a facade, as if the leaders are reading from a script. They sit at the international negotiating tables, such as the World Trade Organisation, but have nothing to negotiate. The seats stay occupied even in the face of meltdown in their societies: the government of Somalia continue to be officially "represented" in the international arena for years after Somalia ceased to have a functioning government in the country itself,"* but ignored the reality of the likely result of investing in a sham (military junta). Did the professor not notice the corrupt "evil genius" as he called himself, at the helm of affairs in Nigeria at the time of SAP? It is my opinion that only people who benefit directly or indirectly from sham governments expect any human economic programme to work by any means other than chance in a shambolic state. SAP during the period of General Babangida could not have been different from the economic policies under Mobutu Sese Seko of Zaire. Nigerians rightly believed, and I share the same belief that these professors were then, and still are basically implementing economic theories not meant for Africa. Without protected industrialisation and a basic level of self-reliance, no ridiculous highfalutin economic programme or strategy will work in Africa. With a market of a billion people, only the current divide and rule prevents the self-sufficiency of Africa. Should the remaining landmass of planet earth somehow become uninhabitable, will mankind not survive and maintain current western living standards in Africa? Besides, who said that economics is a concrete science? I stand happily to be corrected as I go into another man's territory here: *"We don't really care about who owns Daimler, but Africa needs two types of Mercedes Benz - the one manufactured in Africa from scratch and the one imported: The imported ones should cost twice as much as the locally made one."* How about that? The problem of course is the time gap between getting a locally manufactured Mercedes in Africa compared with the imported one. What if we agree to only import vehicles whose manufacturers agree to immediately invest in local production

102

within the AU and slam heavy duties on the rest? This is where having a single market is so important and powerful, even for the poor. What about designer goods and labels? I am sure the Guccis of this world know how Africans love designer goods. How about coming over to one of our SAAs/SARs to begin production from local raw materials and cheap labour? What about helping to build the incomes of the very people you will eventually sell to? Ostentatious goods must be used to finance our manufacturing industry by channelling all proceeds from duties directly into manufacturing only. At least with our SAAs/SARs we will not have the Mugabes (Zimbabwe) Gbagbos (Ivory Coast) and Ratsirakas (Madagascar) of Africa who lose elections and then refuse to hand over power, sabotaging their own economies instead for their own selfish political interests.

The Texas-Africa Cotton Deal

I found myself as the guest of a radio show for the first time ever, talking about Re-Membering Africa. The only telephone caller I was able to respond to asked this question: Why is it that there is an embargo against African goods? She was, like quite a lot of people, very angry about what is generally seen as unfair trade against Africa. Now experts will immediately jump to correct this caller's "ignorance." Of course there is no embargo against African goods. I explained this gently to the caller and gave some hints about a proposed "Texas-Africa Deal" which I will explain shortly. She was not satisfied and called back after the show passionately putting across her views. Conscientious people sense the unfairness of trade when it comes to Africa, and are rightly passionately angry at Western policies for Africa even though they do not understand the true mechanism of the unfairness and propose communist type of solutions. The capitalists on the other hand think they understand the issue better and propose (unbeknownst to them) depraved economic policies with no hope of ever working for Africa's unique situation. What am I talking about? What I am talking about is the subsidies paid to already rich U.S and EU farmers and Africa's reliance on primary commodities. Europe, centuries ago discovered that the middleman owns the market. He basically profits from other people's sweat. By making itself the middleman, Wal-Mart broke the bank, although it would say that it eliminated the middleman. So with Africa not having a middleman economy, she gets her people killed for diamonds and oil while the middlemen elsewhere smile to the bank with the same oil and diamonds. To complicate it further, we simply cannot even productively use these primary commodities as demonstrated by Nigeria's importation of petroleum products and persistent scarcity of such products, despite exporting 2 million barrels of crude oil a day. Is this not simply the result of corruption and incompetence? If Nigeria had an intelligent (free of nepotism and cronyism) petrochemical industry that supplies other African countries and its own domestic market, much more money will be made from the secondary and tertiary products of petroleum. I tried in vain to explain to my passionate radio caller that not until Africa moves beyond its dependence on primary commodities, there will be no significant economic growth for the collective. This is where there is a metaphorical embargo. Moving away from dependence on primary commodities and having some U.S agricultural subsidy abolished, is what the Texas-African Cotton Deal is about. Here is the deal: Oil-rich Texas, like any typical rich person with multiple streams of income will be quick to tell everyone that because one stream of revenue is not very large does not mean that it is dispensable. True, but what if you could actually increase the volume of the stream by taking it somewhere else? Yes, I propose that the subsidy and the American receivers remain exactly the same (meaning that they lose nothing), but with land for farming their cotton shifted into West African SAAs. This is basically a transfer of the subsidy as investments (of the same farmers) into an area with much cheaper labour. Will this not mean a promise of a much higher return on investments of at least 10 times based on the difference in labour costs? Cotton is the best example but other agricultural produce and primary commodities can fit into this model. With this, there will certainly be increased production that will threaten the global price of cotton, but suppose we also plan greater utilization of our cotton in local textile mills in the same SAA? Perhaps here, we can comfortably begin to clothe Candide's Negro with one arm, one leg and rags for clothing. Perhaps instead of second-hand clothes the African clothes market will see more new clothes. Who said that the clothes market is saturated? Is it not time that Africans wear better clothes? This is where the secondary and tertiary markets of cotton and other fabrics come in. Designer clothes makers and big retailers can plan to increase their markets in our SAA using our cheap labour, and for creating the workforce who can afford to buy these clothes, we win twice. I have not suggested that subsidies be abolished immediately. I am only suggesting that a gradual process of shifting it from an area of "selfish concentration" to one of "selfless diffusion" will lead to higher dollar yield, and Texas cotton farmers will see their income grow as they help the international market grow. Arguably the place likely to buy more clothes in the coming years is Africa or any other place where the people move from poverty into middleclass existence.

With this deal, we can anticipate that a lot of subsidies could be removed within 5 years, going at a quasi-experimental rate of 20% diversion of subsidies per year, whilst retaining the lands in Europe and the U.S. Of course, should some catastrophe happen again in Africa that prevents this deal from going on, the previous lands remain. In the meantime, 5 years of investments and greater production should have had the same U.S and EU farmers smiling to the bank with more cash because of more production and consumption. So where is the risk? Farming in current countries that have put in an "embargo" on African farmers by the subsidies paid to their farmers will obviously not stop after subsidies are abolished, but there will then be a global and natural equilibrium. This should be reciprocally beneficial to workers and land owners and farmers with infinite lobbying capacity. Should food security become an issue, rich countries can always re-introduce subsidies. In the interim, so much good would have been done in building the capacities of African farming (not farmers), secondary production and industries. Therefore, let all well-meaning activists and Africa-friendly governments sign up for this deal!

U.S looking for New Course in Africa, says Clinton

I have said it before and I will say it again: Having shown you the blueprint above O Barack, the new course for sustainable U.S. engagement with Africa is in a new AU as a true Pan-African superstate. I have revealed how few people know the real African nationalities, I have explained the issues of incompetent middlemen (unrepresentative governments) and neo-colonialism (exploitation by the middlemen and their foreign collaborators/cold war allies), and I have explained why shambolic states and governments cannot reasonably be expected to deliver sustainable development to the people. Hilary is right; "What happens in Africa has a very direct and growing impact on what happens in Europe and what happens in the United States." No one knows the future, but the best way to predict the future is to create it. Yes, we can write a future history for Africa, for you are in the middle of a biblical prophecy O Barack. Throw the stone O Barack, and the United States of America will have a foothold in the emerging new Africa. Who else but you is better positioned to champion this direction as U.S foreign policy for Africa?

Chapter 4

The Future History of Africa

What is likely to happen once a strong AU or a "United States of Africa" comes into being? How will the Itsekiri people and other small but authentic African nations evolve in this new Utopia? What about representation in sporting events, etc.? There are indeed more questions to ask since no one knows the future. This chapter is my "book of revelations" and like the book of revelations in the bible, all the rather disjointed stories in this chapter have deep meanings. In this chapter, I go a bit into "past history" and it is a means of linking the past to the future. Putting metaphors aside, writing about a "future history" is a bit of a contradiction in terms, but ultimately a statement of deep mystery for those who see visions (young men) and dream dreams (old men) . . . according to the bible that makes it clear that:

And it shall come to pass in the last days, saith God, I will pour out of my Spirit upon all flesh: and your sons and your daughters shall prophesy, and your young men shall see visions, and your old men shall dream dreams - Acts 2:17. Where there is no vision, the people perish: Proverbs 29:18 . . . and my people are destroyed for lack of knowledge: Hosea 4:6

The Truth shall make us free
John 8: 32 . . . and *ye shall know the truth, and the truth shall make you free.*
I begin with this statement because some tribes in Africa may not agree to a strong AU or even to free and fair elections. Why? Because they think they benefit from the status quo. The so-called leaders and elite of the tribe may do, but not the people overall. In reality, no tribe benefits from the 2011 status quo, unless they are very small and their son is in power in a rich country. The Gaddafi tribe

(Muammar Al-Gaddafi's tribe) may be particularly
interested in what I am saying. A member of your tribe
may be in office, but unless you are a close relative, you
are not favoured in any way and will be "sacrificed"
readily in the president or governor's shambolic attempt
to paint a picture of himself as president or governor of
everyone. In reality, all fraudulently elected "leaders" are
there for themselves and not for their tribe, people,
country, conscience or God (otherwise why get in there
by fraud?).

So, how will the authentic, but small and numerous (10,000
according to Martin Meredith) African polities fit into the
huge superstate? I maintain my position that everyone must
have a genuine voice (vote) and seat at the African tribal
house, but, of course not sitting at the same time. The more
groups sitting at the same time, the more unlikely one big tribe
or population group can impose any rule or law not based on
universal positive human values and rights. The practicalities
of the house as far as I can see are no different from the
practicalities of millions of people voting on issues rather than
on personalities. We should have a permanent Festival Town
(or "FESTAC City") in the Central African Republic (CAR),
where thousands of genuine representatives will have the
issues affecting their people constantly in their minds – and
not how to line their wallets as it is in a lot of "parliaments" in
Africa today. Sadly, not very many people may remember the
World African Festival of Arts and Culture since nothing
came after the 1977 extravaganza in Nigeria that left a legacy
in the form of an estate that became a small town within
Lagos. A permanent "legislators' city" can be built creatively
by mixing the display of African culture with the politics of
the continent. How beautiful will this be? With the senate and
tribal houses in this city, we can even expect a university to
naturally spring out from the issues and events that such a
place must generate. If the fear of true democracy hinders our
current unrepresentative "leaders" from immediately going

ahead with building the city, we could at least begin with the cultural elements. Each initial residence (or embassy) of the tribal representative will be built and owned by a polity, tribe or unique group of people including African Diaspora with their own unique cultures. O Barack, how nice will it be to have a piece of Jamaica and the rest of the Caribbean permanently in Africa? Bob Marley's spirit will maintain a permanent presence in there. How pleasant will it be for African Americans to have a permanent piece of Africa, and for Africa to have a permanent presence of African American culture? O Barack, I am talking of the Zion that African Diaspora singers had prophetically seen and sang about. A permanent place for the rich and on-going display of past and evolving African history and culture will be an immediate magnet for tourism and pilgrimage. Why should we not seize such an opportunity? With the full political elements coming in, the African Senate village, embassies of 54 African colonial countries and the rest of the countries of the world can only make the city even more interesting, if not glamorous.

10,000 tribal or ethnic representatives can be shuffled into groups of 10 and only 1000 can seat at a time. If the senate consisting of 200 seats as described earlier do their work very well, basing all laws on principles rather than on parochial interests, then the tribal house is not expected to reject most laws. Besides, if the same "prime-ministers" of the tribe become the only members or part of the "House of Representatives" (lower house of congress) of their respective colonial countries, then they have the unique ability to leverage the strengths of a strong AU to guide weak or improper state laws. Also, because they are genuine representatives of the authentic people with natural patriotism in their hearts, they are expected to be answerable to the monarch and to the people who elected them. If at any local or tribal level there is a special constitutional provision for snap local elections after 6 months of any election, then no group can claim misrepresentation. The prime minister must tell his

109

people how he intends to better their lot. If he fails, then the king or any pressure group from within the tribe can call for the snap election.

I know that some parts of Africa are becoming more and more de-tribalised and de-tribalisation is ultimately the future of mankind as a whole. However, representation by tribe is only an initial means to an end – good, truly representative and accountable government – and not an end in itself. So, who will represent the de-tribalised Africans? Answer: The Senate with its population-based representation. But why should the tribal house have the final say? Answer: So that marginalisation and centuries old inter-ethnic grievances are genuinely addressed by a strong-enough AU. I will now talk about my nation (Itsekiri) and its people (the Itsekiris) because I know my people. I also know that most humans and groups of people have more in common with their perceived rival or enemy than they choose to accept or even realise.

I will digress at this point by stating that I see the Tutsis and Hutus in the Niger Delta and not just in Rwanda and Burundi; this will be made clear in due course. I also believe that I speak for the Cabinda (an exclave of Angola) people of the coast of central Africa. It was in Cabinda that the Togolese national football team bus was attacked during the 2010 African Cup of Nations tournament that Angola hosted and chose a conflict zone as one of its centres. The nations (tribes or kingdoms) in Africa may be small and too numerous in the eyes of colonialist and neo-colonialist (sham governments and their collaborators), but at least they are authentic and virtually all conflicts in Africa can be linked to some form of real or perceived marginalisation or oppression of a tribe or group of people.

The next obvious link to conflict in Africa is natural resources, their exploiters and buyers abroad. An end of armed conflicts in Africa is part of the future history of Africa and only an AU with a common army as a natural peace keeping force can ensure or even enforce genuine peace; but genuine peace is

110

impossible in the absence of justice and fairness. There can be no justice and fairness if the authentic aspirations of the people are simply ignored. By ignoring the existence of the authentic nations and peoples of Africa, and instead favouring a colonial identity and forced colonial geographical entities, the rest of the world makes justice and peace impossible. Now why would any authority or government not support basic honesty, genuine justice and fairness despite the benefits of peace, progress and economic growth? Once again, it is about the benefits for the few and elite who are currently benefitting from dishonesty and the injustices and unfairness in the system. I have already said that this letter is not about abandoning colonial boundaries with immediate effect. These boundaries have become part of our "natural history of social evolution" which cannot and should not be wished away. What we need to understand now is that the environment (external political atmosphere dominated by the gases of colonialism and neo-colonialism) has changed, and that we must direct our social evolution accordingly by allowing the pre-colonial and post-colonial authentic African polities to emerge from hibernation to federate in a pan-African superstate. The existing small states of Africa has produced uneven, but generally small markets and the continent loses out in the magical gestalt that would have resulted, had it been united. What would have become of the state of California had it not been a part of the United States of America and what would the USA have been like without California? The rich parts of Africa simply store and waste their capital abroad to the detriment of the local peoples of a rich land and the continent as a whole. In our new AU, this will be history. What about the situation where a small but rich enclave simply has its own despotic "king" wasting the resources and having fun at the expense of his people? This is already happening with local neo-colonialist, but I have already offered the solution – an English type democratisation of the monarchy with the prime minister of the tribe being democratically elected to the African tribal house. The AU government and

111

common anti-corruption body will not allow the king of a small tribe, nation or country to waste the money of his people. If he is keen on luxuries, then he may invest in the luxuries that our SAAs will provide. No queen would go to France with national carrier for her shopping. Our money will be kept within the system – no *"I pay myself to help you"* type of foreign aid. This is why the strong AU described in chapter 3 is just the beginning.

Now back to the tribe and nation that I know very well. At approximately half a million in number, home and abroad, the Itsekiris form about 0.05% of Africa's one billion people, but this number of people is in the same bracket as the population of Equatorial Guinea and is not too far from Gabon's. As a small but influential tribe in the Niger Delta over the last 500 years, the Itsekiris have been a major player in the region despite being a minority tribe with much larger neighbours. They traded with the Portuguese well before the boom of the slave trade during which they were the major slave traders of the Niger Delta, having villages and settlements dotted along the Benin and Warri rivers – the present day lands of the Itsekiris in dispute with other neighbouring tribes. We have a proud and rich history, a pre-colonial political system of monarchy and a sophisticated system of rights (including the freedom and rights of women) and trade that has left the tribe educated and rich even without the massive petroleum reserve that the Itsekiri nation has. Although few in number, we are virtually everywhere in the globe, but more in Nigeria, the UK and the U.S. In the U.K and the U.S we gather from time to time, dress in our traditional clothing, sing our songs, dance to our music and sing our national anthem and pledge our allegiance to the Olu. Wow! I thought we had moved on since we were colonised over 100 years ago! Even for an educated "Nigerian" married to a "British Arab" how come instead of having Sunday roast, your Arab wife is preparing "igbagba" for the house? The answer: The beauty of multiculturalism and pleasure of an authentic African nationality and culture! If we

112

have this pleasure in Great Britain, why can't we have it in continental Africa?

The average westerner would never have heard of Nana Olomu of the Itsekiris who fought a war with the British. This war, given the might of Britain at the time may be seen as a skirmish, but it was a defining period for the Niger delta. At the time of the war (1894), there was no "Nigeria" and unbeknownst to virtually all Africans, the Berlin Conference had taken place and the Scramble for Africa was on. Nana's dealings with Europeans, like those of Jaja of Opobo make interesting readings. They were savvy capitalists and not nationalists who fought against European imperialism as my fellow "Nigerians" like to portray them. Even as far back as the mid-1860s, there was unfair trade and marginalisation of the majority by the minority (the Itsekiris). The Europeans had their own agenda and the middlemen of the period (the likes of Nana of Itsekiri and Jaja of Opobo) like the middlemen of today (sham governments and despots) collaborated with foreign merchants for their own gains. Indeed, Nana's position as "governor of Benin River," like "Nigeria" of today was a British invention for their imperial and capitalist agenda. It is interesting, almost hilarious to read the histories of "treaties" the British created and signed with whoever they intend to colonise. The Itsekiris or "Jekris" as they were called by the British 100 years ago, prior to British domination had an "Olu" or king and the position remains till today. When in 1894 the British who had without consultation already taken the whole of the Niger Delta as theirs to control, decided to bypass Nana and trade directly with other tribes in the hinterland, Nana "revolted" like the militants in the Niger Delta of today are "revolting" against the Federal "Government" of Nigeria. Nana attacked his fellow traders who were other tribes. The British with their deeper agenda responded in kind by destroying Ebrohimi, Nana's base and sent him on exile. This deeper agenda of the British in early 1897 was to take Lieutenant James Robert Phillips further hinterland to the ancient Benin kingdom where he along with two other British officers and about 200 protectorate forces (allegedly) was killed. A punitive expedition, in line with the deeper agenda followed and the Benin people were massacred in early 1897 by the forces of Rear-Admiral Harry Rawson. The kingdom was burnt down completely, but not before it was looted. Its artefacts and art were carted and sold in Europe and I read in some reports that the money raised officially was "reparations" for killing of Phillips and his men! Some of those artefacts are still in European museums today, although I understand most are held privately and there was an attempt at auctioning a piece for £5 m in late 2010. I take the history of this part of Africa as part of me since I am ¼ Bini by ancestry and grew up in Benin City. I remember when the King of Benin, Oba Akenzua II, died in 1978. Although I was only a 6 year old primary school pupil, I remember the event vividly because the city was gripped with fear of going out at night or being kidnapped and killed as human sacrifice to bury the Oba. Of course the practice of killing slaves to bury a king, which had made Benin City literally a land of blood, was immediately stopped following the Benin massacre of 1897, that did not stop rumours from circulating. So once again we cannot say that colonialism was completely evil, as part of Phillips's ill-fated mission was to ultimately get us to stop some of our horrible cultural practices. Behind the catholic secondary school I attended is the Benin moat – a constant reminder to historically-minded pupils of the defence of the city against invaders. I remember the stories about ghosts in the moat.

It is interesting to see how history repeats itself in many ways! In other words, conflicts in the Niger Delta have never been about the common man, and have had no genuine liberation ideology or moral backing besides the capitalistic chase of material wealth by a few elites. Today, oil is still being traded along the Benin River, not Palm oil, but petroleum. The palm oil that was exported to Europe to lubricate rail lines and used for soap making has now been replaced by the petroleum products used for the fuelling of cars. We can say that

114

arguably, looted oil from the Niger Delta fuels millions of cars in Europe and elsewhere in the world. One of the "freedom fighters" in the Niger Delta, now believed killed by the Nigerian army, was an armed robber and a high school dropout called John Togo. All he really wanted was money as he had not the intellect to understand real political philosophy or the concept of true nationhood, so he picked up his gun. He was given "amnesty" which some see as bribery (in the spirit of "shutting up a few dunces"), but was not satisfied, as indeed he was given a small fish in a mighty ocean of big fishes. Today, the imperialist (neo-colonialist partner of the government/middlemen) is the oil company in the Niger Delta and they cannot stomach disruption of their trade – they either pay up or fight, kill or send on exile the perceived obstacle. In 1995 the dictator and unrestrained thief of national wealth, Sani Abacha found a more innovative way of getting rid of obstacles called judicial murder with a sham trial. Right in the watchful eyes of their neo-colonialist collaborator (the oil company Shell) and during the Commonwealth Heads of Government meeting in Auckland, Abacha executed the playwright, environmentalist and human rights campaigner ken Saro-Wiwa. With the Commonwealth (the remnant of the British Empire) pretending to be a spectator like Shell, I cannot see how Abacha's action was different from those of Rear-Admiral Harry Rawson on the ancient Benin kingdom bringing the might of an empire on a small nation. It is interesting to note that not very many "Nigerians" sympathise with Ken. Why would they? After all Ken is not a "fellow country man" of the majority of Nigerians. He is perceived by some instinctively as attempting to deprive them of "Nigeria's oil" that happens to be underneath his homeland. Some Igbos remember him negatively for supporting the "government" of Nigeria during the barbaric war against Biafra. In reality, ken Saro-Wiwa's Ogoni people were in a forced federation with other nations including Itsekiri, but are too small to have their authentic voice heard in the current British arrangement. If they had gone with the Igbos to form Biafra, the Ogonis still

115

would have remained a small minority in Biafra. Only a pan-African tribal congress can guarantee the rights of the Ogoni people, Igbos and the Itsekiris. Indeed Ken did voice out the nationhood of the Ogoni people and was quickly perceived by parochial minds as making utterances amounting to treason. There is no harm in listening to the authentic African voices, unless to those who wish to perpetuate injustice. Only governing people by their explicit consent can ensure peace in the land and progress of the collective union.

Fellow Itsekiris reading this letter may not accept my portrayal of an Itsekiri national hero and West African historical figure. I apologise in advance for any offence that this may cause, but I will quickly call on the fact that Itsekiris have been Christians for a long time, go back to my statements at the beginning of this last chapter and reach out for my Bible and call on John 8: 32 ... *And ye shall know the truth, and the truth shall make you free.* Given that the Itsekiris can boast of several literary giants of the past and of today, I cannot claim to speak for the Itsekiris. However, I certainly can speak about the Itsekiris from personal experience of what it has been for me to be an Itsekiri of my generation. So what "truth" has the son of Metseagharun for his Itsekiri people? I have said it before, and I'll say it again:

Conflicts in the Niger Coast Protectorate (or Niger Delta) have never been about the common man, and have had no genuine liberation ideology or moral backing besides the capitalistic chase of material wealth by a few elite, until now.
O Barack, all I want to tell you, the world and my people is that some may think that they benefit or hope to benefit from the status quo because a member of the tribe is in position of authority, but in reality only the authentic voice of each nation will bring peace and prosperity to Africa. I did say that I see the Tutsis and Hutus in the Niger Delta and not in Rwanda and Burundi and this is because ethnic tensions, hatred and actual marginalisation has been going on everywhere in Africa including the Niger Delta for centuries. The domination of a majority tribe by a minority tribe is an art of human ingenuity,

116

but ultimately creates a state of injustice and unfairness. This is why Iraq and Bahrain will continue to have tensions for a long time to come, and possibly until the majority express their democratic rights and the minority does not feel threatened. The Itsekiris (a minority tribe) controlled the Benin River and the surrounding areas directly or indirectly for centuries and probably up till the 1950s. Even today, the governor of Delta State is an Itsekiri man. The history of the area is disputed and this is not the medium to go into it, but what cannot be disputed is the animosity that our neighbours held against us for decades for the alleged marginalisation and violation of their rights. Finally in 1997, the pent-up animosity of the Ijaws around the Warri and Benin rivers exploded. The Hutus (Ijaws) went for the Tutsis (Itsekiris) in a war that we thought could only have occurred in the 18th century. Only the fact that the Itsekiris were part of a federation that is much bigger than Rwanda, saved the Itsekiris. Sadly for the Tutsis of Rwanda and Burundi, the strong AU we hope for did not exist in 1994 to save 800,000 and possibly over a million people from being massacred in the worst case of genocide since the 2nd world war. Following the initial Ijaw surprise attacks and "gains" of driving out Itsekiris from most of their villages along the Benin River, Itsekiris took up arms. Again, this is not the medium to go into the gory details of the tragedy, but it is worth noting that beheadings and summary execution took place in the creeks of the Niger Delta, preventing a lot of people from using the water ways. Itsekiris from all over the world gathered to save the nation. A non-Itsekiri friend of mine told me of how he knew the Itsekiris in London had to gather cash for the purchase of weapons to defend the Itsekiri nation. So began the proliferation of small arms in the Niger Delta. So unknown to most people outside the Niger Delta, "rebellion" in the Niger Delta has nothing to do with the environment, Ken Saro-Wiwa, oppression by oil companies, sanctity or other western ideological concepts that are believed to result in war. With war and arms proliferating in a region, what do we know naturally follows in a post-conflict area?

117

Yes, you guessed right; armed robberies and high military or "security" spending. But wait a minute. What else could these armed young men do with these weapons that they now possess in a time of peace? Aha! There is the big fish – the oil companies! Legitimate struggle in the Niger Delta with true understanding of the issues died in 1995 with Ken Saro-Wiwa. I said nothing to my friend who was telling me about Itsekiri self defence initiative, not because I was not aware of the Itsekiri defence efforts, but because I had a deeper, but sad understanding of what was really going on. A year after the Ijaw-Itsekiri crisis started, my father had been murdered by his fellow Itsekiri countrymen. Some of his killers subsequently became "warriors" for the Itsekiri nation. This is the tragedy of a lot of armed rebellion and "armies" in Africa. Those with the guns soon dismiss civil authority and seize the state. The war supposedly ended in 2003, but most Itsekiri villages have failed to thrive since then. Even my home town of Escravos, despite the huge investments in oil exploitation has not recovered. Instead the armed Itsekiri militia have taken over, collecting "rents" from the oil companies and helping to falsify election activities in the area. Another set of our historical middlemen has emerged, posing as representatives of the people whilst at the same time exploiting the people and taking all the available wealth for themselves and close members of their immediate families. With a population of less than a million - a lot of them well-educated - and over 100 oil wells in the Escravos area alone, no Itsekiri is expected to be poor. So where is the money for the people? The simple answer; seized by a few and wasted on frivolities whilst the majority, even for a nation as small as Itsekiri languish in poverty. There is an Equatorial Guinea within the entity called Nigeria. I can say with confidence that the Olu (the Itsekiri king) is rich, but he is not the Nguema of Itsekiri land. However, it is my view that only an elected Itsekiri prime minister, and not a king, may be able to save fellow Itsekiris from themselves. This takes me to the issue of modernising African traditional Institutions. A lot of monarchies besides

118

the Swazi king, are far from absolute monarchies. As a matter of fact, the Nigerian government has the right to depose any traditional ruler. Quite often, like it happened when the British were in charge, monarchs in Nigeria persistently allow themselves to become puppets in the hands of dictators. Some of them and the institution they represent fail to support the people against the vices and exploitation of the federal government, fearing being deposed or side-lined in terms of the benefits that some kings in Nigeria continue to have. So long as the King's hereditary rights are not infringed on, I cannot see why some traditions cannot be modified. Indeed, history by itself modifies all traditions and socially maladaptive traditions that resist modification, soon die naturally any way. As Itsekiris, we have modified our traditions when it was required for adaptation, or simply had change brought in by a punch of knowledge against ignorance and this includes our abandonment of the circumcision of women over 200 years ago, whilst our neighbours continue with the practice. We sadly only eventually abandoned the killing of twins about 50 years ago. With the African Social Security Card and a rig-proof electoral system, we will not have "retired" armed robbers posing as representatives of any local people in a sham rebellion against a sham government. We will have the beauty and benefits of having our leaders from the stock of those with the right head for economic development and not juju worshipers with the wrong psychopathic heart for war, animalistic and biological "survival" instincts, and as a side effect, corruption and thieving. I have already written a vision of Itsekiri 50 years from now coinciding with Nigeria's celebration of 50 years of "independence," so I will not write more about Itsekiri. I have only used the example of my tribe as one of the authentic polities that should form the true African Union, instead of the 54 or more accidents of European history masquerading as "nations," whilst the true neo-colonialist in various forms continue to exploit the people and suppress their authentic voices.

119

It is interesting to read about Shell's espionage activities in Nigeria giving proof to the fact that we have not moved from 150 years ago: The new middlemen in the Niger Coast Protectorate and its trade were the Abachas of Nigeria (ex-presidents). Now that a Christian has become Caesar, what will happen to the Roman Empire of Nigeria? Goodluck Jonathan, the current president of Nigeria, an Ijaw man from a minority tribe in the wider Nigerian context has dodged the issue of a sovereign national conference. He did in fact, expressly dismiss the need or relevance of such a conference, seemingly avowing the sanctity of the 1914 British creation of "Nigeria" as a "sovereign entity." Of course, those from the north of Nigeria can see the king of Kuwait pledging allegiance to Iraq! He has already been accused of harbouring intentions of enabling the Niger Delta to secede from the rest of Nigeria for the obvious gains of shutting off probably about 110 million "leeches" away from the oil wealth of the region. I suppose with this letter to you O Barack, it has become clear that Niger Delta secession will only create an Nguema for the region without the authentic voices of the people. Besides, it will probably make the Itsekiri situation worse as there will be less protection by a big-enough federal government. This is also why a much bigger federal entity in the form of the African superstate will be the best protection for the small and medium sized nations like the entrepreneurial and enterprising Igbos. We already have some budding Nguemas in the Niger Delta as it is today. They are already taking state and local government funds for themselves, stashing our money in foreign banks, and we find ourselves looking up to the British Government to prosecute thieves of state funds and their collaborators on our behalf. With a stronger AU and a pan-African anti-corruption police we will no longer need the British to prosecute our thieves for us. If a stronger AU had been in existence before 2011, South Sudan would never have needed to become a new "country" already engaged in a conflict within itself following a "Yes" outcome of a referendum for independence and killing its own citizens even before it formally declares independence. The reason of course is because South Sudan will be like Nigeria in 1960 – made up of too many tribes. It will not be long before the political entities in an imperfect union begin to fight against each other, having not first clearly agreed on the terms of the union. Getting rid of the colonial or neo-colonial master, common oppressor, enemy or bully is not enough. We do not want South Sudan in the Niger Delta. As a matter for the dynamism of African affairs, a North-South conflict over Abyei has already broken out in Sudan before I could finish writing and editing this letter, O Barack.

Well, I suppose it is politically conducive for Goodluck Jonathan to be very careful especially at the early stages of his presidency . . . but truth is truth! Look at the UAE that had a population of only 95,000 in 1963. Dubai alone is now about 2,000,000 in population and very rich. The possibility of a few becoming extremely rich is not to be feared. What is to be feared is cash moving away from the land. This is the message for Northern Nigeria where some had expressly supported the unpleasant deeds of their fellow northern countrymen who had occupied the position of top middleman (presidency of Nigeria). If a few good people hold the cash on the land, then all smart and hard-working people on the land will benefit. Stagnant cash or cash stashed abroad does nobody any good locally, and the hope of one's relative occupying high office simply perpetuates corruption. All the political thieves in Nigeria both from the North and South have taken money overseas and the local people or tribe actually never really benefitted much from their thieving brother. Even in Western democracies, it is the government and a few who hold most of the money in the country. As I have mentioned already, realistically, only a few people can do certain things requiring high intelligence or expertise. You can choose to vote for a relative, kinsman or a dunce, and he will perform according to his personal interests more than any political philosophy or manifesto. So, genuine democracies tend to "even out" into a pyramid (water finds its own level) where the majority at the

121

bottom find themselves voting for the minority at the top if they are to have their intellectually-challenging problems genuinely solved. If we choose to vote for an incompetent person purely because he is our tribesman or because he is poor like the rest of us, then what made him incompetent or poor may be shared with the rest of us. We don't want that. However, the reality of democracy is sometimes that the minority in the form of moneybags simply directly or indirectly buy their way to power. In sad cases, a minority in the form of a group of proper thieves (minority, because the majority cannot be proper thieves by default) simply steals power! What we want is to have the minority in the form of the intellectually-sound and politically competent to deliver all the good that the minority has for the majority, even though this tends not to be realistic for the obvious reason that water finds its own level, and a natural pyramid of abilities and of people most often springs out. So, even with democracy, aristocracy must find its way to the top, otherwise the majority suffer the consequences. The problem with so-called democracy in Africa is that quite often votes are sold, offices are bought and a criminal usually successfully emerges as "leader" of the people in a sham state. In our new AU, meritocracy will reign and everyone with a heart for fairness will benefit from it.

Seeing tomorrow:
"How good and how pleasant it would be, before God and man to see the unification of all Africans?" – Bob Marley 1979, Survival
Dear Dr Temi, I thought I'd send you a card to say thank you for the help you have given me recently. I know its "just in a day's work" for you but I want to remind you that your work changes lives for the better, mine included!
Kind regards, D.G

African & Development studies undergraduate,
University of XXXXX

Above is the near-exact writing of a patient on a thank you card. I encountered him in the course of my work as a psychiatrist; not as a philosopher or political scientist. He sent me a card just before he left for Africa. He was going for an initial stint as part of his undergraduate career, but vowed to live permanently in Africa. I thought I knew about the philosophy of Bob Marley and the spirit behind his songs, but I didn't and so I was prompted to check out the rest of the lyrics.

> *As it's been said already, let it be done, yeah! As it's been said already, let it be done, yeah!*
> - *Bob Marley*

Soon I realised that *"We are all African"* is not just a cliché! Bob Marley prophetically saw the unification of all Africans and where else can we all unite if not in the landmass of Africa? He did sing about "Rastaman" and "higher man" and did not necessarily mean "all black people" even though in our prejudiced minds "African" always conjures up a black-skinned individual. These are part of the problems of human boundaries that some humans thankfully have now transcended. It is not about race or colour or even the nationalities created by man. We are all mixed races! We are of one spirit and this is what D.G and I shared. He could not wait to go back to Africa to serve. Oh, by the way, D.G is completely white-skinned, blonde-haired and raised in the UK. All Africans uniting means the whole of mankind uniting to accelerate the political and socio-economic integration of the continent; to promote and defend African common positions on issues of interest to the continent and its peoples; to achieve peace and security in Africa; and to promote democratic institutions, good governance and human rights - The very aims and objectives of the AU as it stands today. So-
Africa unite:
'Cause the children (Africa unite) wanna come home.
Africa unite:
'Cause we're moving right out of Babylon, yea,

And we're grooving to our Father's land, yea-ea.

How good and how pleasant it would be before God and man
    So-o: Africa unite,
    Afri - Africa unite, yeah!
    Unite for the benefit (Africa unite) for the benefit of your
    people!
    Unite for it's later (Africa unite) than you think!
    Unite for the benefit (Africa unite) of my children!
    Unite for it's later (Africa uniting) than you think!
    Africa awaits (Africa unite) its creators!
    Africa awaiting (Africa uniting) its Creator!
    Africa, you're my (Africa unite) forefather cornerstone!
    Unite for the Africans (Africa uniting) abroad
    Unite for the Africans (Africa unite) a yard! *[fadeout]*

O Barack Obama, we cannot sing in a letter or book, but
the spirit had been in the air for decades for Africa to
unite. Most of the "countries" of Africa now in existence
in the year 2011 were created by people living outside of
Africa, and sadly must be helped by people living outside
of Africa. Those of us Africans left behind on the soil of
Africa by our boundaries creators were left on our own to
pick up the pieces of the Berlin Conference and get on
with "nation building" without recognition of our true
nationalities! Independence turned out to be half a century
of farce! I, along with the Itsekiri people was made British
in 1885 and I have never had, and never sought
independence. Our so-called "nationalists" realised their
error within a decade of the colonial masters leaving, and
by the 3rd and 4th decade saw our delusional independence
in the form of home-grown neo-colonialism. Some of
them saw it in their graves and others in jail. This is not
fair and explains why foreign aid has not worked so far. It
is difficult to build a nation that is not yours and you have
no true allegiance to. Our new AU beginning with the
SAAs and SARs will reduce the impact of the economic

124

sabotage and corruption of sham states and government on the people. O Barack, it is about the people, not the "states" or their "governments". The more we focus on the people the more the states and government improve.

2007 AD
A black president of the U.S? No . . . no, no, not in our lifetime.
Well, that was the voice of the pessimist silenced by history and in your person O Barack.

2011 AD
A truly united Africa? Well, let's wait and see, but how marvellous and pleasant will it be before God and man to see a superstate created with the fundamental positive and universal human rights and values in its foundation? Suppose that superstate is called Africa?

How marvellous and pleasant it would be before God and man to see the cradle of civilization burst back into life with the ancient and modern side by side! Ancient Africa's best product is mankind as a whole. The history of our evolution and migration from Africa is told in our genes. In *Dreams from my Father*, you were right Barack in quoting William Faulkner, that *the past is never dead. It's not even past.* Over-flogging our colonial past and victimhood is not the aim of this letter, but we cannot move from or set aside our past if we have no genuine alternative future history (vision) to make our future, O Barack. I say once again that this writing is not a thesis rich in facts, literature and the bibliography of an academic, but we are reminded once again of Faulkner that *so vast, so limitless in capacity is man's imagination to disperse and burn away the rubble-dross of fact and probability, leaving only truth and dream. Remember me, says Africa. Put my dismembered parts together O Barack.* You cannot afford to allow this opportunity to unite Africa pass you and us by . . . .

125

YOU WILL REMEMBER ME.

THE END